LOW CARB ON THE GO

More than 80 fast, healthy

recipes—anytime, anywhere

LOW CARB ON THE GO

More than 80 fast, healthy recipes—anytime, anywhere

Text and photography by
Sandra and Mirco Stupning

PREFACE

6

INTRODUCTION

8

BREAKFAST

20

BREADS AND SPREADS

52

CONTENTS

VEGETARIAN

80

MEAT
AND FISH

126

SNACKS
AND CAKES

158

INDEX

186

CONTENTS

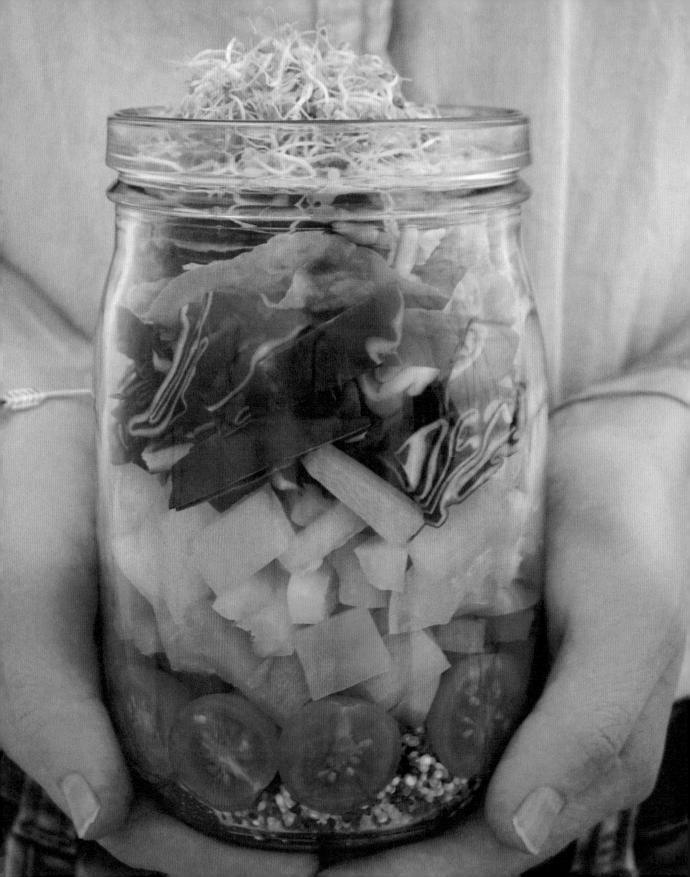

PREFACE

We are delighted that you want to prepare delicious low-carb dishes to take with you when you're out and about. We are often asked what is the easiest way to stick to a low-carb diet during lunch breaks or when traveling, especially since it is rare to find any low-carb carry-out options at your local sandwich counter. Our solution: prepare food at home and take it with you.

Our delicious and healthy low-carb recipes can be quickly prepared at home and the finishing touches added at work in just a few minutes. And if you have delicious ready-made food packed up for your lunch break, you won't be tempted to go and grab something else from the cafeteria, bakery, or supermarket. Enjoy using this book and take our healthy recipes as a source of inspiration. There is no need to follow our suggestions exactly as we have described them. Creativity and using your own favorite ingredients are invariably the best ways to ensure you have fun in the kitchen and that the food you make really is to your taste.

And remember, eating with others is always better than sitting alone at the table. Turn your lunch break into a communal experience. It is not just eating that is more enjoyable as a group. Why not do the preparation together, too? Arranging a lunch date is not unusual, but an even better idea is to meet up in the kitchen to get the food ready. It is often much easier to stick to resolutions as a group and therefore achieve preset goals, such as eating a healthier diet. With several people to help, salads can be rustled up in no time. The food and ingredients can be agreed on in advance and everyone can bring something with them, or you can take turns with your colleagues when dishes need to be prepared at home.

Our low-carb recipes will support your healthy lifestyle and boost vitality. Have lots of fun with our dishes to go.

Best wishes
SANDRA & MIRCO STUPNING

Low carb doesn't mean no carb!

The aim of a low-carb diet is to reduce, as far as possible, your consumption of poor-quality foods that are high in carbohydrates and focus instead on alternative options and healthy carbohydrates. It isn't a question of avoiding all carbohydrates; indeed, it isn't healthy for the human body to be denied carbohydrates altogether long term. If carbohydrate intake is drastically restricted, the body has to adjust to generate energy in some other way. In addition, an extreme reduction in carbohydrate consumption can have a negative impact on our health because the body is deprived of numerous important substances, particularly if this diet is followed over a long period. This kind of radical dietary change should only be done under medical supervision. If you want to slim down in a healthy way, you need to expend more energy than you consume, and that is best achieved through a healthy diet and exercise. The number of carbohydrates eaten should always be adjusted depending on how much physical exercise you are doing. A sensible approach is to eat fewer carbohydrates on days when you are relatively inactive than on days when you have workouts lined up. Creating a meal plan is highly recommended when losing weight.

WHAT ROLE DO CARBOHYDRATES PLAY IN THE BODY?

Carbohydrates are our most important source of energy. They are needed to generate energy in the body's cells and they serve as fuel, an energy storage system, and a basic framework for our DNA and RNA, which carry our genetic information. If the body doesn't need all the energy that is provided by a meal, it converts any excess into fat stores. A diet that is low in carbohydrates, ideally combined with several exercise sessions each week, allows the body to break down any excess fat.

But the low-carb diet is not just a good choice if you wish to lose weight. Plenty of health-conscious people tend toward this lifestyle because of the focus on a varied and balanced diet and, in particular, because it avoids too many pasta products, baked goods, and highly processed or ready-made foods. Instead the emphasis is on vegetables, salads, fruits, nuts, seeds, and good-quality fats. It is not a question of banning foods, but rather of placing the emphasis on choosing the right foods.

"GOOD" AND "BAD" CARBOHYDRATES

Carbohydrates vary in composition. The more complex the structure of the carbohydrate consumed, the longer the body needs to break it down and process it. The body has to break carbohydrates down into simple sugars before they can be absorbed into the bloodstream. This breakdown process, to convert molecular chains into their constituents, requires energy.

THE BUILDING BLOCKS

The basic building blocks of carbohydrates are monosaccharides (or simple sugars). In their smallest unit, these consist of a single sugar molecule. Disaccharides, as the name suggests, consist of two monosaccharides joined together. Longer, partly branching sugar chains are described as oligosaccharides or polysaccharides.

Monosaccharide (simple sugars)	Disaccharide (double sugars)	Oligosaccharide (complex sugars)	Polysaccharide (complex sugars)
1 single sugar molecule	2 linked monosaccharides	3 –10 linked monosaccharides	> 10 linked monosaccharides
glucose, fructose, galactose	sucrose, maltose, lactose	raffinose, stachyose, verbascose	starch, pectin, cellulose, glycogen

GOOD CARBOHYDRATES are complex carbohydrates. They consist of lots of individual sugar molecules, which are chemically bonded together in chains and are subdivided into oligosaccharides and polysaccharides. They are found, for example, in vegetables, fruits, nuts, whole grains, and soy. The body needs longer to break down these carbohydrates, so blood sugar levels rise only slightly, the body does not produce much insulin, and the danger of storing fat in the body is low. Complex carbohydrates make you feel full for longer because the energy obtained from them remains in the body for longer. That is why eating complex carbohydrates is recommended for losing weight.

BAD CARBOHYDRATES are simple carbohydrates, which are easy to absorb. These are processed quickly by the body and enter the bloodstream swiftly. These monosaccharides and disaccharides are primarily found in processed foods containing refined sugar and white extra-fine flour. They include confectionery, pastries and pasta made from inferior-quality flour, various pre-prepared meals, fast foods, potato chips, soft drinks, and alcoholic beverages. Simple carbohydrates are broken down swiftly by the body and don't make you feel full for long. Hunger pangs are the inevitable result.

Sugar in the blood

The most important sugar circulating in our blood is glucose – a monosaccharide. All carbohydrate compounds contained in food are broken down into individual sugar molecules by the body and can only be used once this has been done. The brain, our red blood cells, and our kidneys all rely on glucose. All other somatic cells obtain their energy primarily by metabolizing dietary fats.

The body needs more time to break down long, branching carbohydrate compounds than it does for simple compounds. This is why complex carbohydrates make us feel full for longer and allow our blood sugar levels to rise and fall gently. The reason this is important is because wild fluctuations in blood sugar levels (a blood sugar roller coaster) cause food cravings and lapses in concentration. If blood sugar levels are constantly careening up and down, the consequence can be obesity and diabetes.

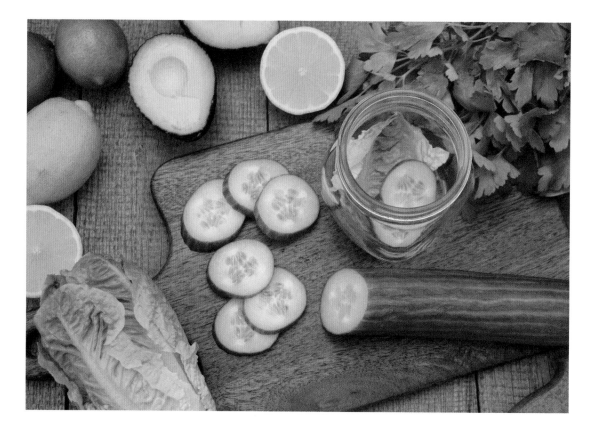

WHAT CAUSES A BLOOD SUGAR ROLLER COASTER?

All sugar chains are broken down in the digestive organs. The resulting small sugar molecules then penetrate the cell walls and are absorbed into the blood and the blood sugar level rises. As a consequence of the rising sugar level, the brain receives a signal that the body is full and insulin is released from the pancreas. The hormone insulin allows sugar to penetrate into cells and be used as a fuel.

As soon as the sugar in our bloodstream has been absorbed by our cells, the blood sugar level falls again and the brain receives a signal that the body is hungry. At this point we often reach for something to eat again, especially sweet things (blood sugar response 1, see right). If the body is constantly exposed to this roller coaster, this creates stress. The elevated insulin production causes a strain on the pancreas, which can result in pancreatic malfunction. In addition, the body may become resistant to insulin.

HOW CAN THIS BE AVOIDED?

It is better to eat carbohydrates that are complex in structure, with vegetables and salads at the top of the list. Legumes, such as beans, lentils, and peas; "activated" nuts (which have been soaked in water); whole grains such as spelt; and pseudo grains such as buckwheat also all deliver slowly digestible carbohydrates. These foods prevent blood sugar levels from rising and falling too rapidly (blood sugar response 2, see below). The dietary fiber contained in complex carbohydrates also ensures a well-regulated digestive system.

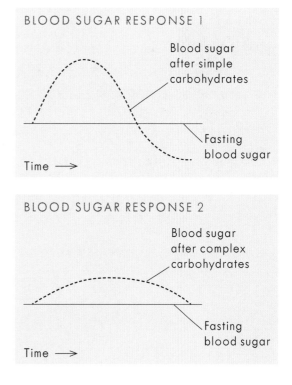

BLOOD SUGAR RESPONSE 1

Blood sugar after simple carbohydrates

Fasting blood sugar

Time ⟶

BLOOD SUGAR RESPONSE 2

Blood sugar after complex carbohydrates

Fasting blood sugar

Time ⟶

Healthy carbohydrate consumption during the day

A daily consumption of 100–150 grams of carbohydrates is ideal for the human body. The brain and nervous system require around 120 grams of carbohydrates each day; they cannot obtain energy from fats and so are dependent on glucose. If consumption is too low, the body has to take over glucose production (gluconeogenesis) itself in order to guarantee an energy supply for these organs. This isn't healthy in the long run because if you avoid carbohydrates completely, you would no longer have a balanced diet. Eating too much protein, meat, and fish is not a good foundation for a fit and healthy body. We recommend sufficient consumption of healthy carbohydrates such as vegetables and fruits, which, along with healthy carbohydrates, also contain vital nutrients and fiber.

HOW MANY MEALS SHOULD I EAT DAILY?

It is highly recommended to limit yourself to three main meals a day. This is because our digestive system functions best if we avoid constantly bombarding it with new food on top of the contents of the last meal while it is still being processed in the digestive tract, even if the additional food is just fruits, vegetables, or a wholesome snack bar. In particular, if you are trying to lose weight, it makes sense to avoid snacks as far as possible. At first, this may be really hard to stick to. Our tip: if you get hungry between meals, a glass of noncarbonated water can sometimes help. Often it is not really hunger, but just thirst, food cravings, or simply habit that prompt us to start snacking.

If you really do need something to eat between meals, especially when you are initially changing over to a low-carb diet, you should stick to healthy snacks. In the morning you can chop up some fruit, or a low-carb bar is another good option. Both of these will provide energy and satisfy your cravings until the next meal, and are better than a snack containing rapidly absorbed carbohydrates such as white flour or sugar. Vegetables and nuts are suitable snacks at any time of day. Even low-carb baked goods, such as biscuits, muffins, or waffles, are great to have with you occasionally to nibble on. Other easily prepared snacks include cheese cubes, hard-boiled eggs, olives, or berries.

For each of our recipes, the carbohydrate content is specified in grams. This makes it easy to plan your total carbohydrate consumption each day. The summary also specifies how many portions each recipe makes.

MORNING

Breakfast is the time when most carbohydrates should be consumed. This is because the body requires energy after its overnight rest. We recommend a portion of good carbohydrates, perhaps from a smoothie; some yogurt—plain or with berries; a serving of fruits, nuts, and seeds; some low-carb muesli; or low-carb bread. Since fruit is digested quickest, eat it first to avoid having it sitting on top of foodstuffs that take much longer to digest. At breakfast, you should consume between 40 and 70 grams of complex carbohydrates.

MIDDAY

It is vital to make vegetables a major component of your lunchtime meal. Lots of different salads provide an ideal source of good carbohydrates. In small quantities, beans, lentils, and peas, but also quinoa and low-carb noodles, can enhance the midday meal with complex carbohydrates and important nutrients. Fruits should mainly be consumed during the first half of the day and should form a smaller proportion of your intake than vegetables. For your midday meal, eat between 40 and 50 grams of carbohydrates.

EVENING

At the end of the day, the body is generally winding down and needs only a small amount of energy in the form of carbohydrates, so just a small quantity of carbohydrates should be eaten at this

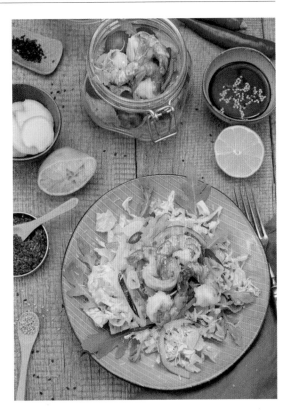

point. Salads and vegetables, along with a good portion of protein, are ideal. Healthy sources of protein include eggs, nuts, seeds, and also mushrooms. If you opt for animal protein at dinner time, you can enjoy some fish, shellfish, cheese, or meat. However, meat should not be eaten too late, as the body needs several hours to digest it. Fish, on the other hand, is easier to digest and will pass through the digestive system within an hour. The recommended carbohydrate intake for the evening is no more than 30 grams.

The low carb exchange

DON'T EAT THIS	EAT THIS
pasta made from wheat or durum wheat semolina	vegetables, low-carb noodles, whole-grain noodles in small quantities
white rice	riced cauliflower, brown rice in small quantities
potatoes	vegetables
French fries	oven-baked sweet potato or zucchini
bread and rolls	low-carb bread and rolls
burger buns	"oopsies" low-carb buns (see p68)
pizza	pizza with a cauliflower or low-carb flour base, low-carb pizza
white flour	flours made from nuts, linseed, coconut, hemp, chia, sesame seed or soy, whole grains
wraps	lettuce leaves, spinach wraps, omelets
breaded fish and meat	fish and meat without a breadcrumb coating
nuggets and other reconstituted fish and meat products	a single cut of fish or meat— ideally organic
pre-prepared meals, baking and sauce mixes	freshly prepared dishes
milk	plant-based "milks" such as almond, soy, oat, and coconut
premade muesli and breakfast cereals	homemade muesli
soft drinks	water with fresh fruits
juices	spritzers with fresh juice, tea

DON'T EAT THIS	EAT THIS
store-bought ice cream	homemade fruit ice cream
sweets	frozen berries and dried fruits
muesli bars	low-carb bars
cakes and cookies	cakes and cookies made from low-carb flours and nuts
chocolate high in sugar and with a low cocoa content	cocoa nibs, dark chocolate with a high cocoa content
chocolates and confectionery	homemade pralines from dates and nuts
latte and macchiato	coffee without milk
sugar	coconut sugar, honey, agave syrup, low-calorie sweetener such as stevia

CHOOSE RAW NOW AND AGAIN

There are lots of benefits to eating foods raw rather than boiling, frying, or baking them. All the active ingredients are preserved and are available to our bodies in their natural form.

The most important substances in vegetables, salads, and fruits are vitamins, minerals, secondary plant substances such as glucosides, and fiber. Raw fruits and vegetables also contain enzymes. Our body requires enzymes, minerals, and vitamins for all the metabolic processes in its cells. Secondary plant substances and fiber help promote healthy digestion.

As a consequence, eating lettuce, vegetables, and fruits in their raw form is highly recommended. The greater the variety of plant-based foods consumed, the greater the range of substances obtained as a result.

Basic equipment for transporting meals

Delicious packed meals definitely require the right containers for transportation. Various sizes of glass jars with screw caps (twist-off jars) or a snap-close fastening are ideal for taking meals with you. Not only are colorfully filled jars aesthetically pleasing, they are also airtight and won't leak. Glass doesn't absorb flavors and can be filled with hot liquids without any problem. We also use circular and rectangular containers with click-to-lock fasteners.

TEST FOR LEAKS

If you don't want to buy jars especially for storage, you can reuse food jars and containers like the ones that once contained yogurt or jam. The most practical containers have a wide opening to make it easy to add ingredients to your meal.

Whatever kind of jar you choose, you should always test it in advance to make sure it doesn't leak. To do this, simply fill the jar with water, close it, and then stand it upside down for several minutes. Also make sure the lid doesn't open up too easily when being transported in a bag. If the jar passes the test, soak it in a tub of water for a few hours (ideally overnight) so that the label is easy to remove.

CLEAN AND SAFE

Glass jars should be sterilized before use. You can do this by washing them and putting them, without their lid, in an oven at 350°F (180°C) for around 10 minutes, then switch off the appliance and leave the jars to cool in the closed oven. Alternatively, wash the jars and boil them for 10 minutes in a large saucepan before leaving them to cool down on a kitchen towel. Then the jars are ready for use. Sterilization is important for jars in which jams or spreads will be stored for long periods in the refrigerator. If the dish is going to be eaten promptly, it is sufficient to wash the jar before use, ideally in the dishwasher.

ALTERNATIVES TO GLASS

Unfortunately, carrying glass jars is not always permitted. For example, lots of schools and nurseries prohibit glass containers for safety reasons. The best solution is to use a container or box made from a nontoxic material. You can also get transparent, shatterproof, odor-neutral containers that are free from harmful bisphenol A (BPA). We explicitly advise against using aluminum foil for packaging, as it can contaminate food with a alarming level of aluminum—acidic foods in particular can cause the aluminum to leach rapidly from the foil.

Icons in the book

Various icons are included on each recipe page. The icons indicate at a glance which utensils and equipment need to be taken with you for preparing the dish later at work.

	Containers: ideally glass			Hotplate or burner: saucepan or frying pan
	Kettle			Cutlery: metal, wood, or even chopsticks
	Jars: large and small			Oven

WARM DISHES bring variety to your breaks. Some low-carb dishes can be eaten warm or cold as desired. We prefer to heat dishes in the oven or on the stove top. Alternatively, you can use a microwave.

THE PREPARATION TIME is subdivided into the time required at home for preparation plus baking, soaking, and so on, and the time which you will need later at work to finish preparing the dish.

NUTRITIONAL VALUES per portion are also provided in table form. The nutritional information always relates to one portion of the dish, and the figures are rounded up or down to the nearest whole number.

Selecting and preparing ingredients

High-quality foods guarantee the most enjoyment. So from the moment you go shopping, you should be focused on getting top-quality, fresh produce. Our preference is to use organic ingredients.

SALAD LEAVES
should always be allowed to drain thoroughly after washing, or ideally dried using a salad spinner, as this keeps the leaves fresh and crunchy for longer.

BEANS, PEAS
and other canned foods must always be rinsed and allowed to drain thoroughly in a strainer.

EGG YOLK OR EGG WHITE
that isn't used can be kept for other dishes, such as omelets, pancakes, or low-carb baked items.

CUCUMBER SEEDS
release water, so remove them before taking this ingredient with you. The seeds can be used in smoothies.

HERBS
stay fresher and are more aromatic if they are chopped just before consumption.

MILK
in our recipes is usually replaced by plant-based alternatives: almond, soy, or coconut milk.

OIL
should only be added to the dish just before eating, as salad leaves in particular go mushy very quickly and won't look at all appetizing.

YOGURT
should not be low fat, because higher-fat products have a slightly lower proportion of carbohydrates than those with a low fat content; some featured are plant-based alternatives, such as unsweetened natural soy yogurt.

SALT
draws water from food, and so should only be added shortly before eating. We like to use sea salt.

BEAN SPROUTS AND OTHER SHOOTS
should always be rinsed thoroughly and allowed to drain in a strainer or on paper towels.

SWEETENERS
made from natural ingredients are our preferred option. These include agave syrup, coconut sugar, honey, and dates. If you would prefer to avoid carbohydrates altogether in your sugar, use a low-calorie sweetener extracted from plants, such as stevia.

LEMON AND LIME JUICE
are always freshly squeezed—we keep these fruits on hand at all times, ready to be squeezed.

Layering your jar

To ensure your food stays fresh and crisp until lunchtime, it is best to stick to a certain order: heavy ingredients, such as beans or cabbage, go into the jar first, which prevents lighter ingredients from being crushed. Foods that release juice, such as carrots or oranges, and ingredients that are prepared with liquid, such as quinoa, should also go into the jar first. This ensures any moisture remains at the bottom and doesn't run through all the other ingredients. Next come vegetables, then fruits, then salad. After this you can put in any meat, fish, or cheese, The uppermost layer consists of the topping, such as nuts, seeds, superfoods, or shoots, which add the finishing touch to your jar. The jar must seal tightly and be leakproof.

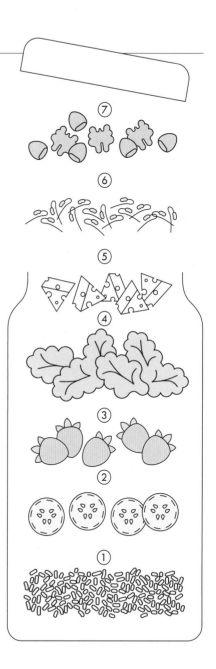

SEQUENCE IN THE JAR

1. Quinoa, pasta, beans
2. Vegetables
3. Fruits
4. Salad
5. Cheese, meat, fish
6. Sprouts and shoots
7. Nuts, seeds

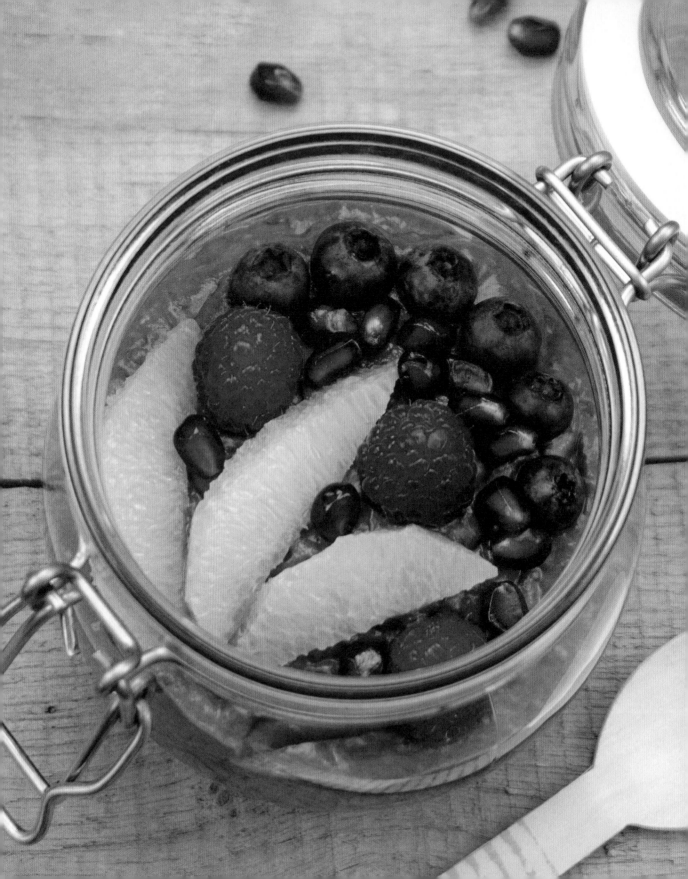

BREAKFAST

Almond milk
homemade

5½oz (150g) almonds
½ tsp lemon juice
seeds from 1 vanilla pod
pinch of salt

Wash the almonds and place them in a bowl. Cover the almonds completely with water, then add the lemon juice. Cover the bowl with plastic wrap and leave the almonds to soak for at least 8 hours, or ideally overnight.

Drain the almonds in a sieve and rinse them again. Place the almonds, vanilla seeds, and salt in a food processor, add 14fl oz (400ml) water, and blend until the ingredients form a fine, creamy liquid. Place a large sieve over a bowl and line it with a muslin cloth. Strain the almond liquid through the cloth, doing this in several batches. If any mixture remains in the cloth, gather the corners of the cloth together above the mixture and twist firmly to squeeze the mixture out.

Pour the almond mixture into a glass bottle and seal. The almond milk can be stored in the refrigerator for 2–3 days. Before using, shake the bottle well to disperse the layer of fat that will have formed on the surface.

OUR TIP—You can make your own almond flour from the leftover almond purée. To do this, spread the almond mixture on a baking sheet lined with parchment paper and leave to dry in a non-fan-assisted oven at around 175°F (80°C). Transfer the mixture to a food processor and blend until it is finely ground. Store the flour in the refrigerator.

At home	At work	Makes	Kcal	Protein	Carbs	Fat
20 mins + 8 hrs	0 min	12fl oz (350ml)	26	1g	1g	2g

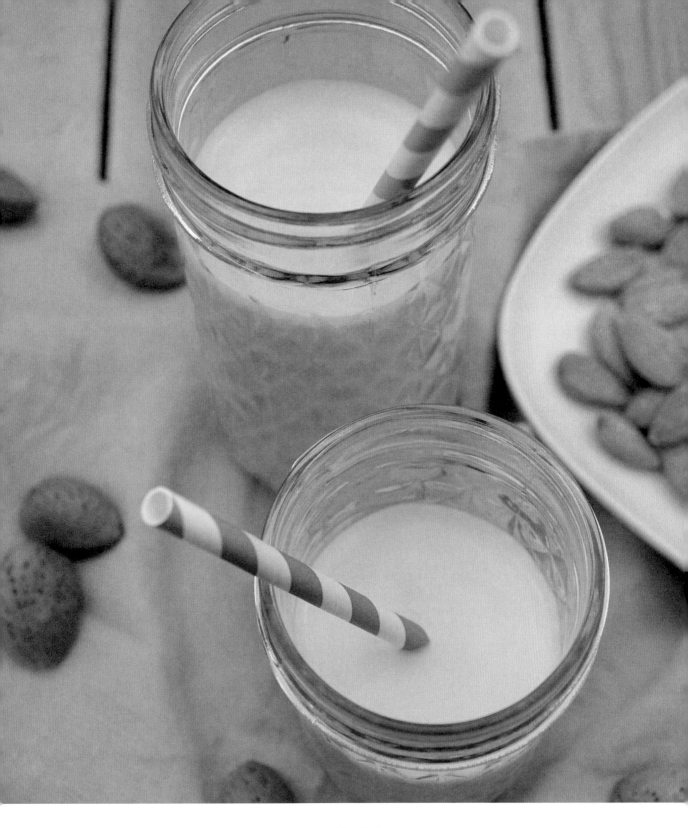

Chocolate smoothie
with avocado

½ avocado, pitted
7fl oz (200ml) almond milk
  (see p. 22, or store-bought)
1oz (30g) banana, frozen
  if desired
2 tbsp raw cocoa powder
2 tsp agave syrup
cocoa nibs (optional)

Scoop out the flesh from the avocado and place in a food processor with the almond milk, banana, cocoa, and agave syrup. Blend until smooth. If necessary, add a little water to obtain the desired consistency. Pour the smoothie into a jar and seal. Store in the refrigerator until ready to drink.

AT WORK—Garnish the smoothie with cocoa nibs, if desired.

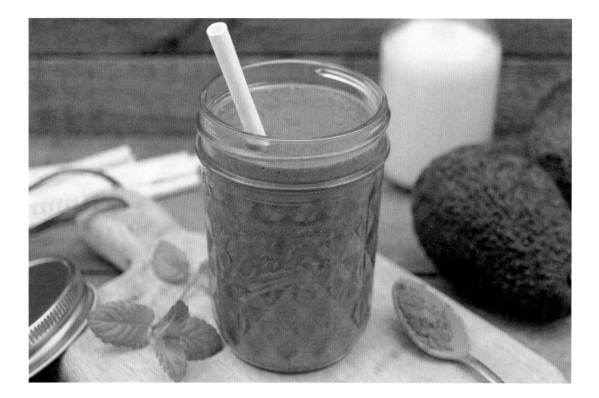

At home	At work	Serves	Kcal	Protein	Carbs	Fat
5 mins	1 min	1	317	7g	14g	20g

Strawberry chia smoothie

with almond milk

2½oz (75g) strawberries, hulled
1 tbsp yogurt
5½fl oz (160ml) almond milk
    (see p. 22, or store-bought)
sliced strawberries for garnish
    (optional)
1 tbsp chia seeds

Place the strawberries, yogurt, and almond milk in a food processor and blend to a fine consistency. Pour the smoothie into a jar, adding sliced strawberries as garnish, if desired. Seal the jar and store in the refrigerator until ready to drink. Store the chia seeds in a separate container.

AT WORK—Add the chia seeds to the smoothie and shake well. Drink the smoothie immediately, as the swelling chia seeds will alter the consistency dramatically.

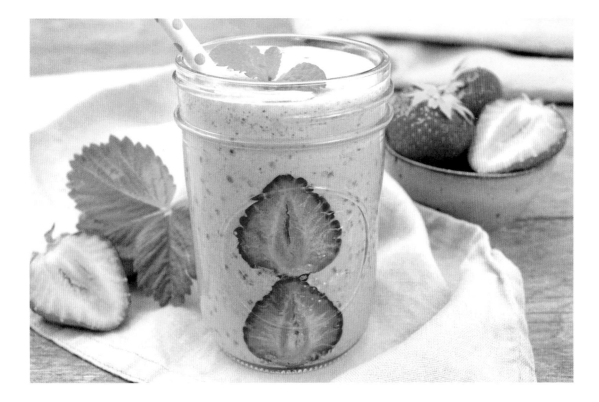

At home	At work	Serves	Kcal	Protein	Carbs	Fat
5 mins	1 min	1	107	4g	6g	6g

Cucumber shake
with dill

5½oz (150g) cucumber, chopped
4 sprigs of dill
½ small apple, cored and
   roughly chopped
3½fl oz (100ml) buttermilk
3½fl oz (100ml) soy milk
pinch of salt and freshly ground
   black pepper

Place the cucumber, dill, and apple in a food processor. Add the buttermilk, soy milk, and seasoning and blend to a fine consistency. Pour the cucumber shake into a glass bottle and seal. Store in the refrigerator until ready to drink.

AT WORK—Pour the shake into a glass to drink.

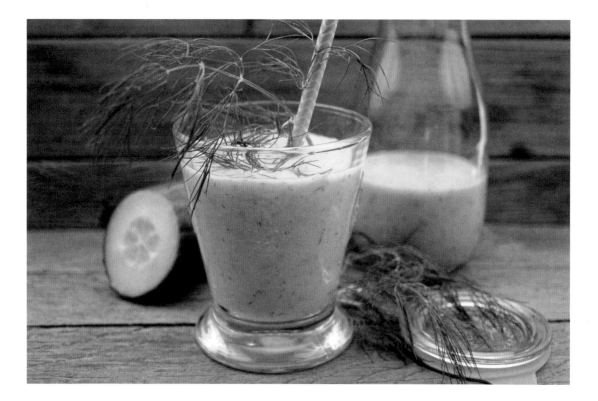

At home	At work	Serves	Kcal	Protein	Carbs	Fat
5 mins	0 min	1	135	8g	16g	4g

Orange shake
with buttermilk

4½fl oz (130ml) buttermilk
2¾fl oz (85ml) almond milk (see p. 22, or store-bought)
1 orange, peeled and divided into segments
1 banana, peeled and chopped

Place the buttermilk, almond milk, orange segments, and banana pieces in a food processor and blend thoroughly. Pour the orange shake into a glass bottle and seal. Store the shake in the refrigerator until ready to drink.

AT WORK—Decant the shake into a glass to drink.

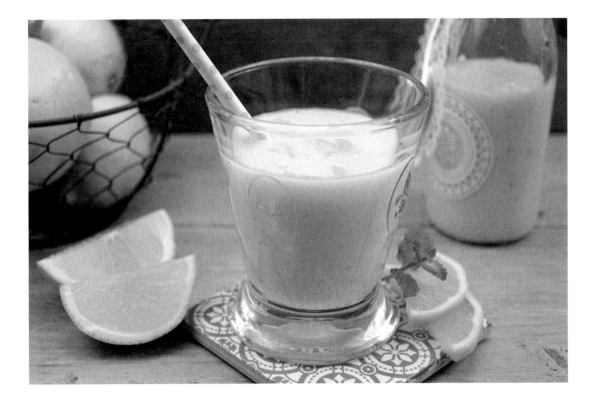

At home	At work	Serves	Kcal	Protein	Carbs	Fat
5 mins	0 min	1	173	7g	28g	3g

Mango lassi

with vanilla

½ mango, peeled, pitted, and
    cut into chunks
seeds from ½ vanilla pod
2½oz (75g) yogurt
5fl oz (150ml) almond milk
    (see p. 22, or store-bought)
1 tbsp lemon juice

Place the mango in a blender beaker along with the vanilla seeds, yogurt, almond milk, and lemon juice. Blend everything thoroughly using a hand-held blender. Pour the mango lassi into a glass bottle and put the lid on. Store in the refrigerator until ready to drink.

AT WORK—Transfer the lassi into a glass to drink.

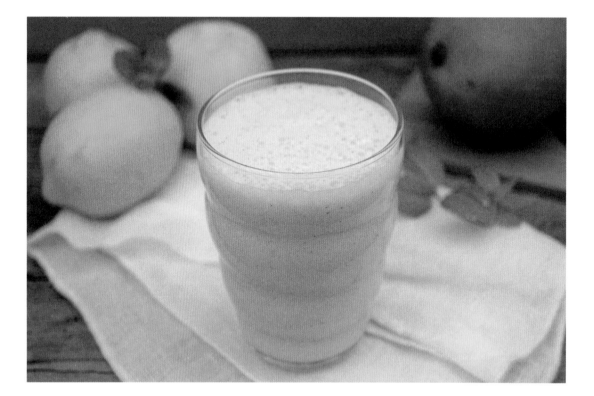

At home	At work	Serves	Kcal	Protein	Carbs	Fat
5 mins	0 min	1	136	5g	15g	4g

Mandarin citrus drink

refreshingly fruity

---

1 orange, divided into segments
juice of 3 mandarins
1 tbsp lemon juice

Place the orange segments in a blender beaker along with the mandarin and lemon juice. Add 7fl oz (200ml) water and blend until smooth. Pour into a jar and seal with the lid.

OUR TIP—Depending on the time of year, this can be enjoyed either as a cold refreshment or heated for a warming drink.

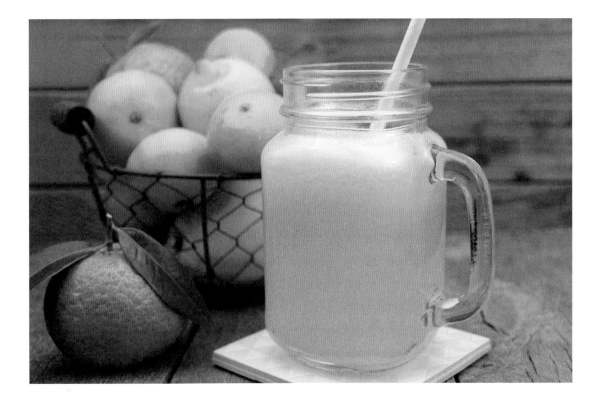

At home	At work	Serves	Kcal	Protein	Carbs	Fat
5 mins	0 min	1	80	1g	16g	0g

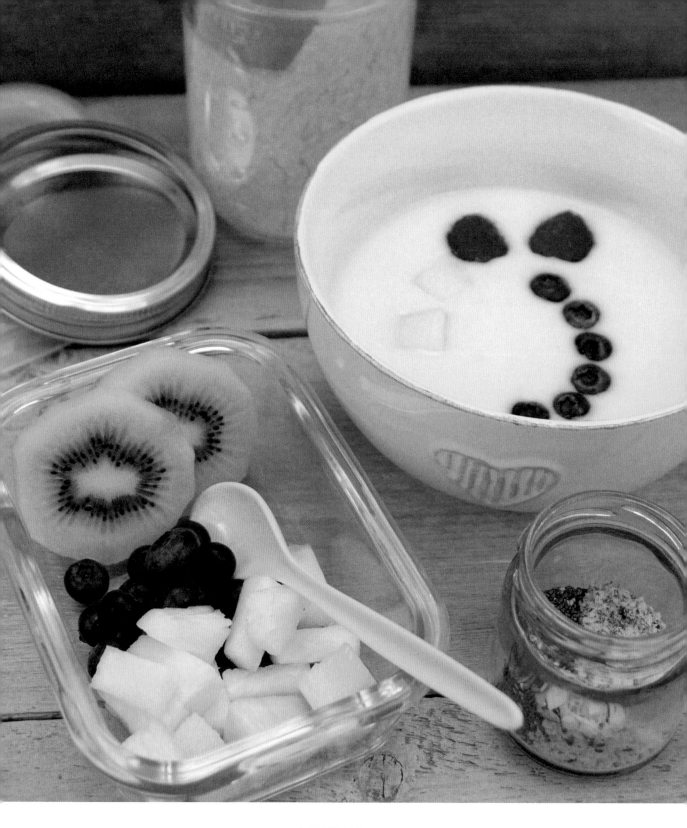

BREAKFAST

Coconut bowl
piña colada style

FOR THE SMOOTHIE
3½oz (100g) pineapple, peeled,
    cored, and chopped
3½ tbsp coconut milk
4 tbsp yogurt
agave syrup (optional)

FOR THE TOPPING
2 raspberries
1 tbsp blueberries
1 tbsp pineapple pieces
2 slices of kiwi
2 small pieces of mango
1 tsp chia seeds
1 tsp coconut flakes
2 tbsp ground almonds
edible flowers, for example,
    violets (optional)

To make the smoothie, place the pineapple pieces in a food processor with the coconut milk and yogurt and blend until smooth. If desired, sweeten the smoothie with agave syrup, then quickly blend everything together again.

To remove the pineapple fibers, strain the smoothie through a sieve into an airtight jar and seal. Store the smoothie in the refrigerator until ready to drink.

Put all the fruit for the topping into a container, then put the chia seeds, coconut flakes, ground almonds, and edible flowers, if using, in a separate container.

AT WORK—Pour the smoothie into a bowl and decorate with the topping ingredients.

At home	At work	Serves	Kcal	Protein	Carbs	Fat
10 mins	5 mins	1	415	12g	25g	27g

Green smoothie bowl
with goji berries

FOR THE SMOOTHIE
½ avocado, pitted
1¾oz (50g) spinach leaves, coarse stems removed
1oz (30g) banana, frozen

FOR THE TOPPING
1 tsp goji berries, chopped
1 tsp blueberries
1 small piece of avocado
1 small piece of banana
2 spinach leaves (optional)
½ tsp white sesame seeds

For the smoothie, scrape the flesh from the avocado skin using a spoon. Place the spinach, avocado, banana, and 3½fl oz (100ml) water in a food processor and blend until smooth. Pour the smoothie into an airtight container and seal. Store in the refrigerator until ready to serve.

Put all the ingredients for the topping into a separate container.

AT WORK—Pour the smoothie into a bowl, then scatter on the ingredients for the topping.

OUR TIP—The topping looks particularly decorative if you cut stars or other shapes out of the avocado and banana, or even from the spinach leaves, if you prefer.

At home	At work	Serves	Kcal	Protein	Carbs	Fat
10 mins	2 mins	1	175	3g	13g	11g

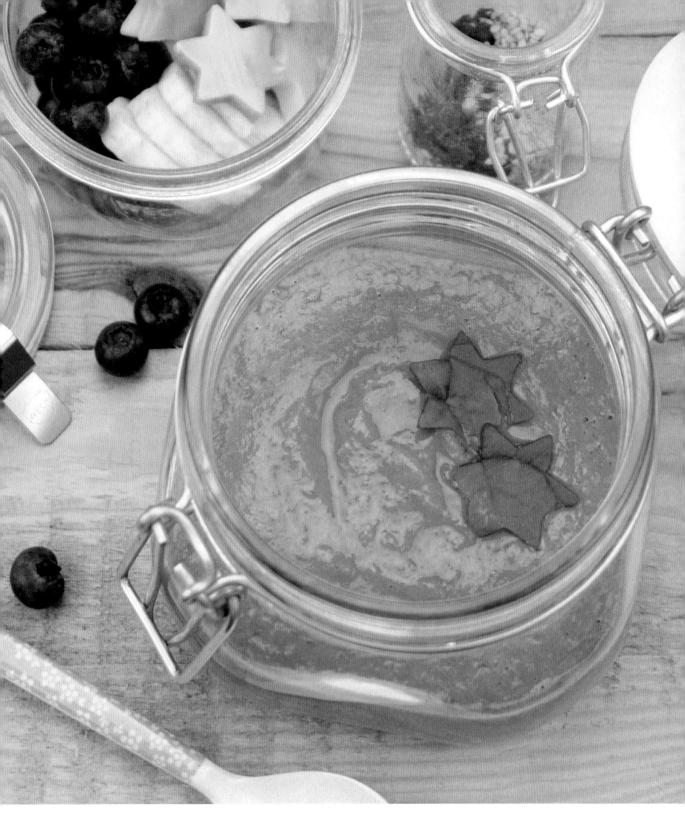

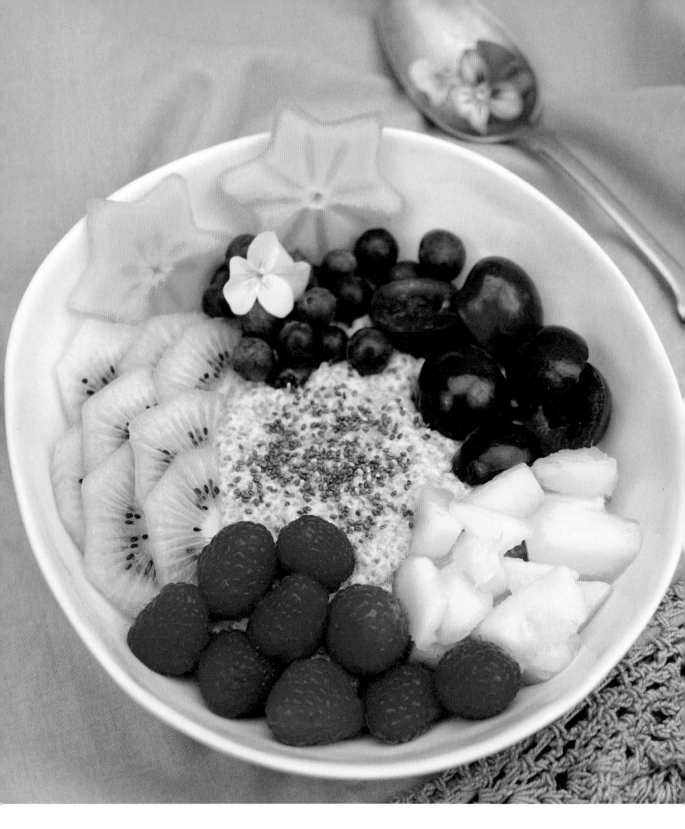

BREAKFAST

Chia breakfast bowl
with fruit

FOR THE BREAKFAST BOWL
¾oz (20g) chia seeds
3½fl oz (100ml) coconut milk

FOR THE TOPPING
2 tbsp raspberries
2 tbsp blueberries
1 kiwi, peeled and sliced
3 sweet cherries, pitted
   and halved
¼ persimmon, peeled and sliced,
   or cut into star shapes
1 tbsp mango pieces
edible flowers, for example,
   violets (optional)

To make the breakfast bowl, combine the chia seeds with the coconut milk in a bowl and leave to swell.

Transfer the chia mixture into an airtight container and seal. Put the fruits for the topping into a separate container. Store the chia mixture, fruits, and edible flowers (if using) in the refrigerator until ready to serve.

AT WORK—Pour the chia mixture into a bowl and decorate with the fruit topping and edible flowers, if desired.

At home	At work	Serves	Kcal	Protein	Carbs	Fat
15 mins	1 min	1	385	7g	22g	26g

Choco chia bowl
with fruit

FOR THE SMOOTHIE
½ avocado, pitted
¾oz (20g) banana, frozen
2 tbsp raw cocoa powder
1 tbsp chia seeds
1–2 tsp agave syrup
3½fl oz (100ml) almond milk
  (see p. 22, or store-bought)

FOR THE TOPPING
¼ orange, peeled and divided
  into segments
1 tbsp blueberries
1 tbsp raspberries
1 tbsp pomegranate seeds
mint or lemon balm leaves
  (optional)

Scrape out the flesh from the avocado skin using a spoon.

Place the avocado flesh in a food processor, along with the banana, cocoa powder, chia seeds, agave syrup, and almond milk and blend everything until smooth. If required, add a little water to obtain the desired consistency. Transfer the smoothie to an airtight container and seal. Store in the refrigerator until ready to serve.

For the topping, put the orange segments, blueberries, raspberries, and pomegranate seeds in a container and, if using, put the mint or lemon balm leaves into a separate container.

AT WORK—Transfer the choco chia smoothie into a bowl and decorate with the topping. Garnish with mint or lemon balm leaves, if desired.

At home	At work	Serves	Kcal	Protein	Carbs	Fat
5 mins	2 mins	1	445	12g	19g	34g

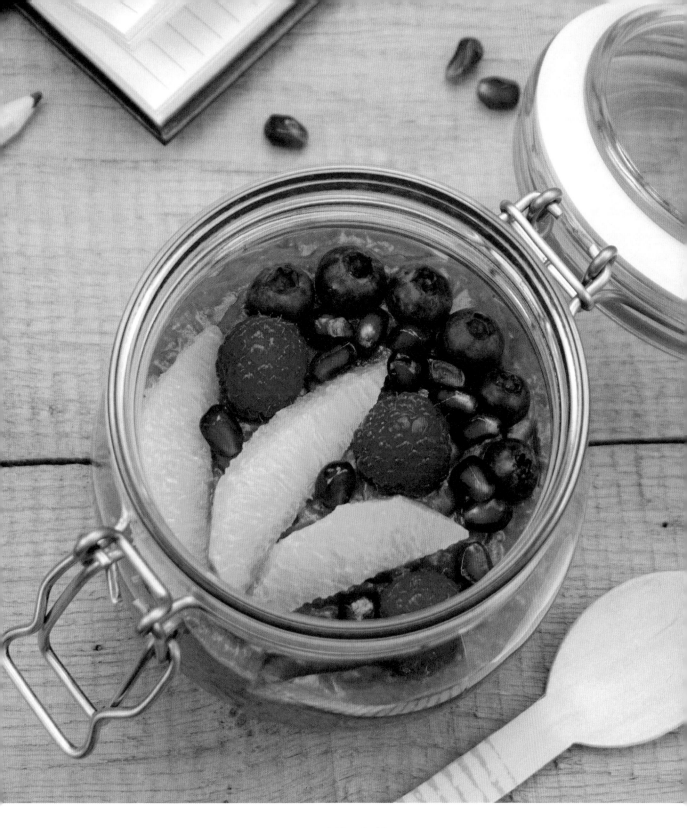

BREAKFAST

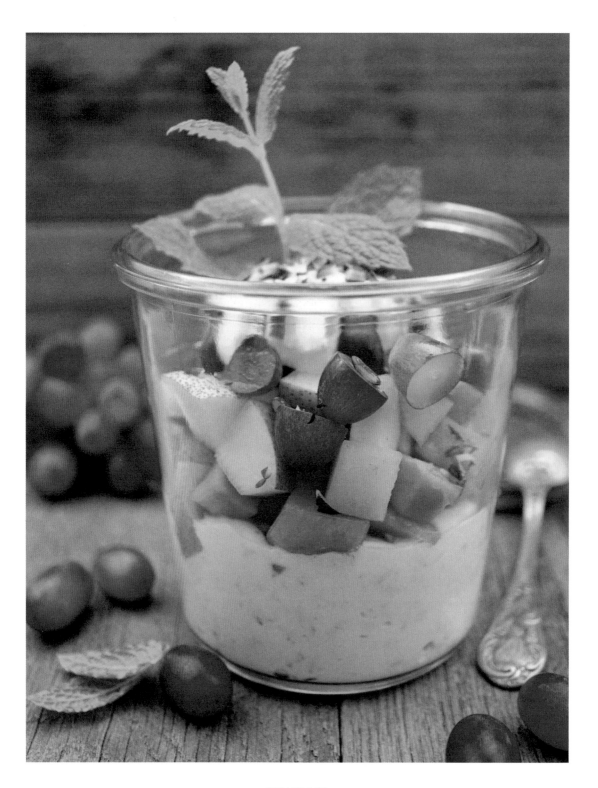

BREAKFAST

Papaya pear yogurt
with pumpkin seeds

5½oz (150g) plain Greek
   yogurt (thick)
1 tbsp spelt flakes
1 tbsp mint, chopped
2½oz (75g) papaya, cored and
   chopped into bite-size pieces
¼ pear, cored and cut into cubes
handful of grapes (red or white,
   as preferred), halved
1 tbsp pumpkin seeds, coarsely
   chopped
sprig of mint, to garnish (optional)

Place the Greek yogurt, spelt flakes, and mint together in a bowl and stir until combined.

Put the mixture into a jar, setting aside 1 tablespoon for decoration. Layer the papaya, pear, and grapes on top. Add a blob of the remaining yogurt mixture and scatter with the pumpkin seeds. Garnish with the sprig of mint, if desired. Place the lid on the jar and store the papaya and pear yogurt in the refrigerator until ready to serve.

At home	At work	Serves	Kcal	Protein	Carbs	Fat
5 mins	0 min	1	314	19g	29g	13g

Lime mandarin yogurt

with superfoods

FOR THE CHIA GEL

1 tsp ground dried dandelion
   leaves (available from
   health-food stores)
1 tbsp chia seeds
1 tsp mint, chopped
1–2 tsp agave syrup

FOR THE YOGURT

juice and zest of 1 organic
   lime, plus slice of lime, to
   garnish (optional)
9oz (250g) plain Greek
   yogurt (thick)
juice of 1 mandarin
dash of agave syrup

FOR THE SUPERFOOD
TOPPING

½ tsp sunflower seeds
½ tsp goji berries
½ tsp pumpkin seeds
½ tsp cocoa nibs
½ tsp hemp seeds
½ tsp pistachio kernels

To make the chia gel, place 3½fl oz (100ml) water, 2 tbsp of lime juice from the yogurt mixture, and the dandelion leaves in a bowl and stir to combine. Mix in the chia seeds and leave to swell for at least 10 minutes. Stir in the mint and agave syrup.

In a separate bowl, stir together the Greek yogurt, the remaining lime juice, and the mandarin juice. Mix in the grated lime zest and agave syrup.

To make the superfood topping, roughly chop all the ingredients, then mix them together in a bowl. Transfer the chia gel to a jar, add the yogurt mixture and, if desired, garnish with a slice of lime. Finally, top with the chopped superfoods. Place the lid on the jar and store in the refrigerator until ready to serve.

At home	At work	Serves	Kcal	Protein	Carbs	Fat
20 mins	0 min	1	435	29g	29g	21g

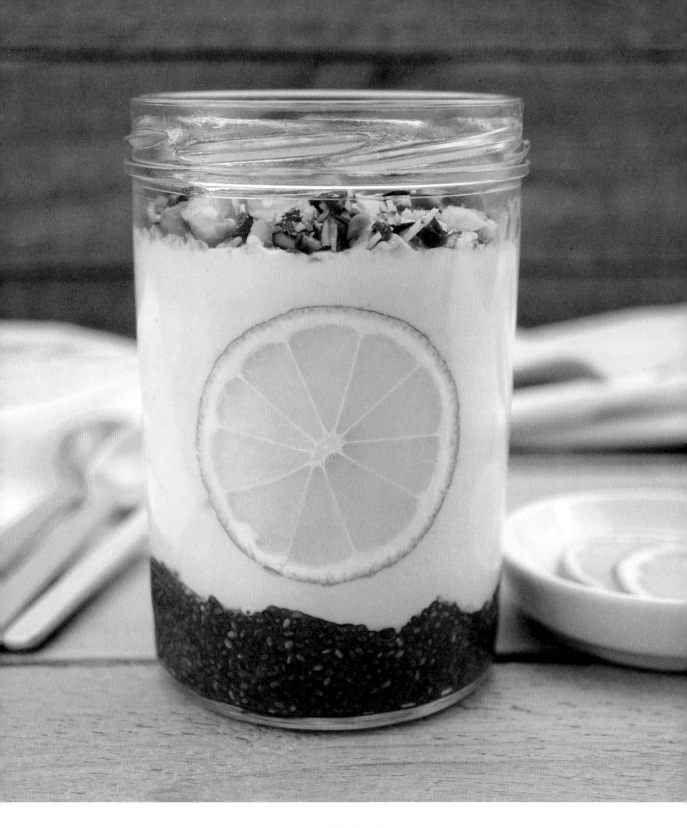

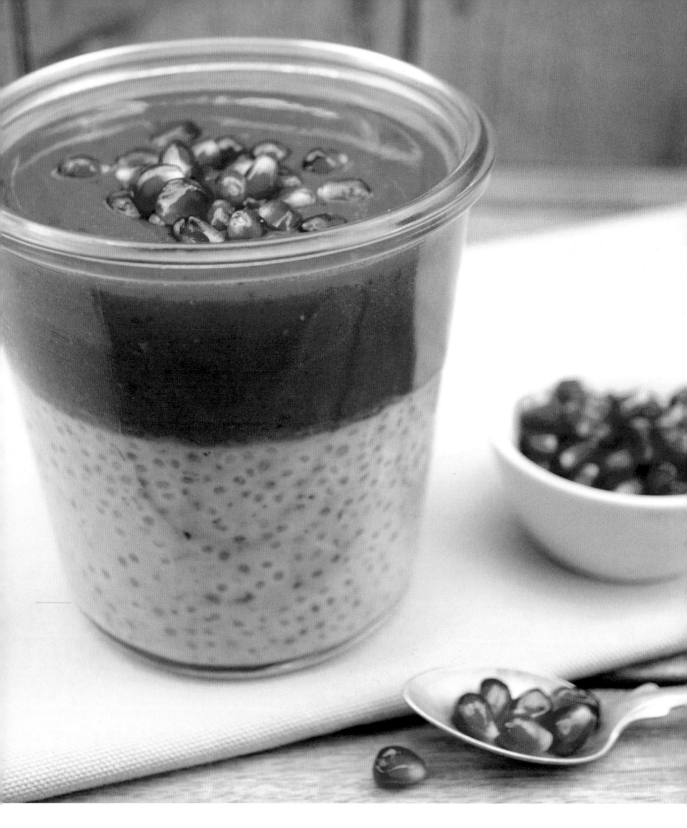

Chia pudding with berry purée
and pomegranate seeds

1 tbsp chia seeds
5½oz (150g) mixed berries (fresh or frozen)
1 tbsp low-calorie sweetener, such as stevia
7oz (200g) yogurt
1 tbsp pomegranate seeds

Mix the chia seeds with 4½fl oz (130ml) water in a bowl and leave to swell for at least 10 minutes, creating a chia gel. Purée the berries in a high-sided container using a hand-held blender (there is no need to defrost frozen berries).

Stir the sweetener into the yogurt. Combine the yogurt mixture with the chia gel, stirring well.

Transfer the chia pudding to a jar. Top with the berry purée and scatter with pomegranate seeds. Place the lid on the jar and store the chia dessert in the refrigerator until ready to serve.

At home	At work	Serves	Kcal	Protein	Carbs	Fat
15 mins	0 min	1	260	12g	18g	9g

Yogurt muesli

with melon

1 tbsp oats
3½oz (100g) yogurt
3½oz (100g) plain Greek
  yogurt (thick)
½ small apple, cored and
  chopped into bite-size chunks
1 orange, peeled, divided into
  segments, then chopped into
  small pieces
2oz (60g) Galia melon, flesh
  removed and chopped into
  bite-size chunks
1 tbsp linseed
1 tsp cashews, roughly chopped

Place the oats in a bowl with 2 tbsp water, stir, and leave to soak for 5–10 minutes, then pour out any excess water. Stir the yogurt and Greek yogurt into the oats.

Combine all the fruit pieces in a bowl with the linseed and cashew nuts.

Transfer the yogurt and Greek yogurt mixture into an airtight jar and arrange the fruit on top. Place the lid on the jar and store the muesli in the refrigerator until ready to serve.

At home	At work	Serves	Kcal	Protein	Carbs	Fat
10 mins	0 min	1	298	18g	25g	13g

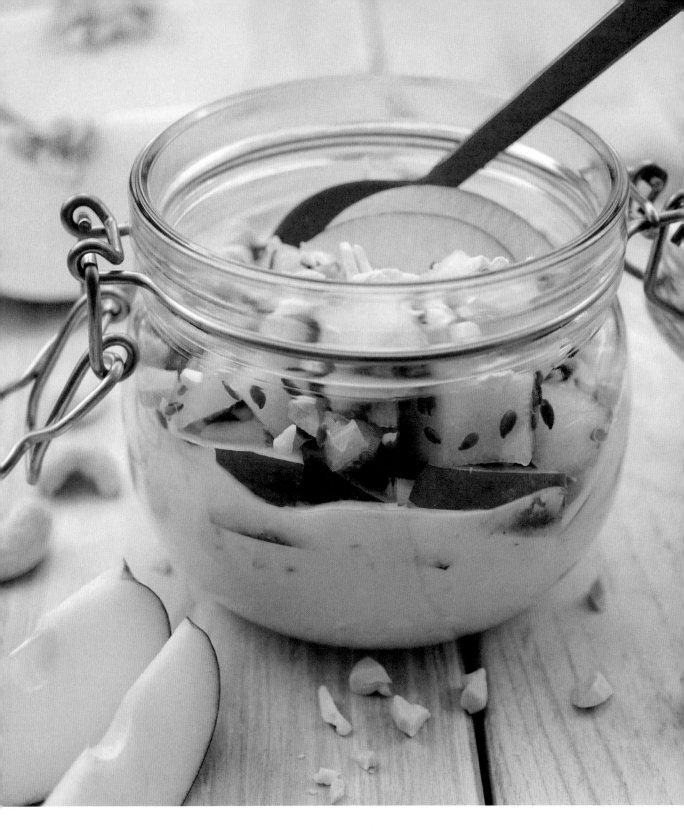

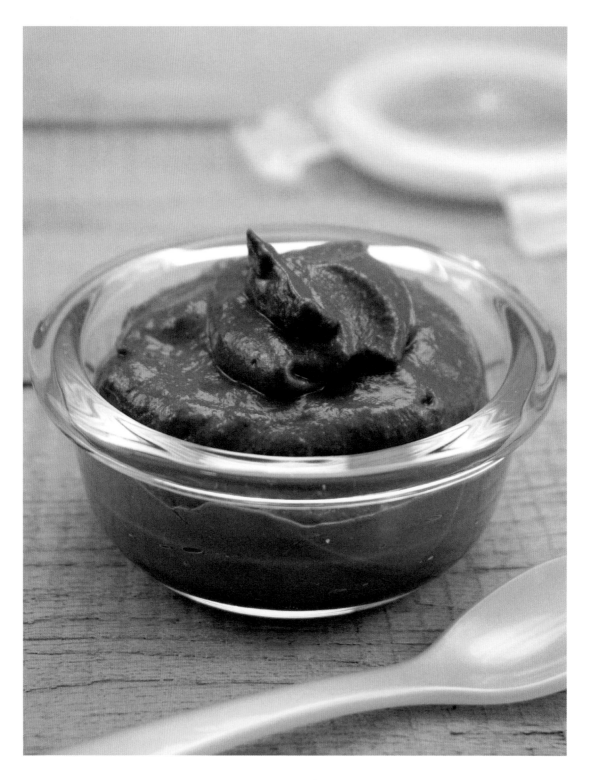

BREAKFAST

Chocolate pudding

extra creamy

---

1 avocado, halved and pitted
½oz (15g) raw cocoa powder
2 dates, pitted
2½fl oz (80ml) almond milk
   (see p. 22, or store-bought)

Use a spoon to scoop the flesh from the avocado skin, then add to a high-sided blender beaker along with the cocoa powder, dates, and almond milk.

Use a hand-held blender to purée the pudding ingredients to a fine and creamy consistency. Transfer to a lidded jar. Store the pudding in the refrigerator until ready to serve.

At home	At work	Serves	Kcal	Protein	Carbs	Fat
5 mins	0 min	1	314	6g	9g	28g

Strawberry bowl
with avocado

1 avocado, halved and pitted
1 tsp lime juice
2 tsp chia seeds
2oz (60g) strawberries, hulled
3oz (85g) yogurt
1oz (30g) mango

Peel one half of the avocado and slice into strips, then drizzle with the lime juice. Put the avocado slices, chia seeds, and 1 strawberry into separate containers. Scrape the remaining avocado flesh from the skin and blend in a food processor with the remaining strawberries, the yogurt, and the mango until the mix is a fine consistency. Store in a container in the refrigerator.

AT WORK—Transfer the mixture into a bowl and garnish with the avocado slices, strawberries, and chia seeds.

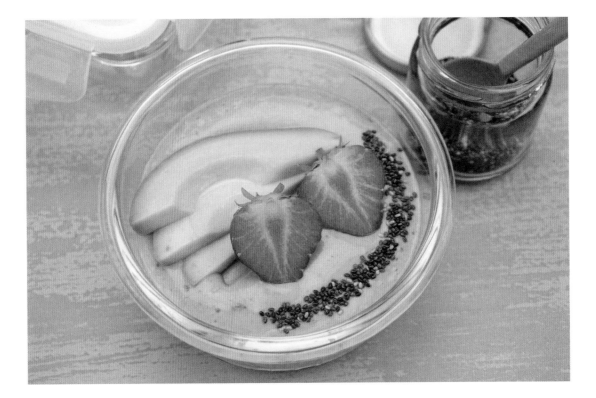

At home	At work	Serves	Kcal	Protein	Carbs	Fat
5 mins	1 min	1	405	8g	10g	35g

Chia pick-me-up
with turmeric

2 tbsp chia seeds, plus a few
  more, to garnish
3½fl oz (100 ml) soy milk
1¾oz (50g) plain Greek yogurt
  (thick), plus 1 tbsp, to garnish
1 tsp ground turmeric
1 tbsp lemon juice
dash of agave syrup
½ kiwi, peeled and sliced

Place the chia seeds and soy milk in a bowl, stir, and leave
the seeds to swell for at least 10 minutes. Stir in the Greek
yogurt, turmeric, lemon juice, and agave syrup. Transfer the chia
dessert to a jar, adding some whole kiwi slices as desired and
setting aside the remaining slices. Garnish with 1 tbsp Greek
yogurt and a few chia seeds. Halve the remaining kiwi slices and
stick them into the top. Seal the jar and store your pick-me-up
in the refrigerator until required.

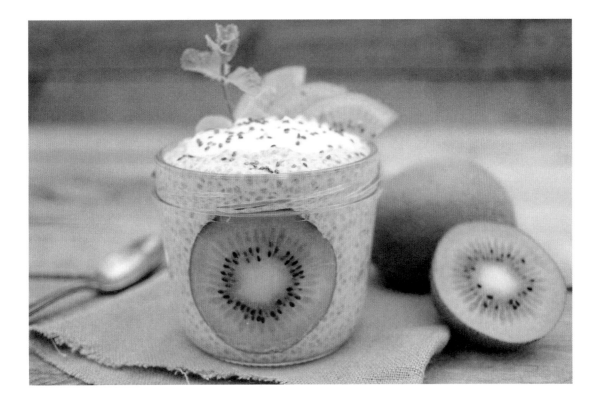

At home	At work	Serves	Kcal	Protein	Carbs	Fat
15 mins	0 min	1	394	15g	13g	24g

Coconut muesli

with a crunch

3½oz (100g) coconut flakes
1oz (30g) sunflower seeds
1¾oz (50g) chopped almonds
1 scant oz (25g) walnuts, chopped
1 scant oz (25g) coconut flour
2 egg whites
1 tbsp protein powder (coconut)
1 tsp low-calorie sweetener,
    such as stevia

Preheat the oven to 250°F (130°C). Line a baking sheet with parchment paper. Mix all the ingredients with 4 tsp water. Spread the mixture over the parchment paper and bake in the center of the oven for 20–30 minutes, until pale gold in color, stirring the mixture two or three times during this period. Remove from the oven, leave to cool, and store in an airtight jar.

OUR TIP—This coconut muesli tastes fantastic with almond milk (see p. 22).

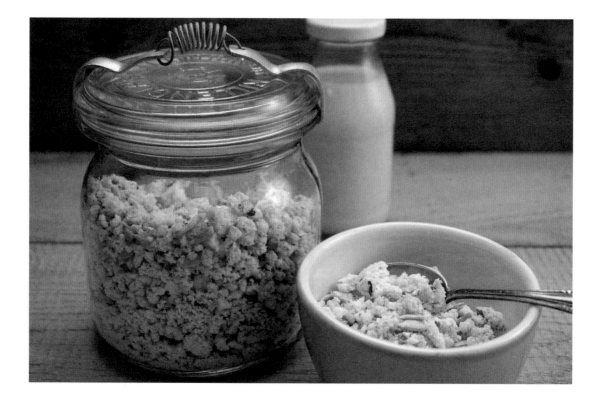

At home	At work	Serves	Kcal	Protein	Carbs	Fat
40 mins	0 min	6	240	8g	5g	20g

Revitalizing muesli
nutty and wholesome

1 tbsp coconut oil
1½ tbsp honey
¾oz (20g) flaked almonds
1 scant oz (25g) oats
¼oz (10g) coconut flour
¼oz (10g) ground almonds
½ tsp vanilla powder (or seeds from ½ vanilla pod)
pinch of salt

Preheat the oven to 275°F (140°C). Line a baking sheet with parchment paper. Melt the oil with the honey in a pan over low heat. Crumble the flaked almonds and combine with the oats, coconut flour, ground almonds, vanilla, salt, and the oil mixture. Bake the muesli on the sheet in the center of the oven for 10 minutes. Reduce the temperature to 210°F (100°C), stir the muesli, and bake 5–10 minutes longer, until golden brown. Leave to cool and store in an airtight jar.

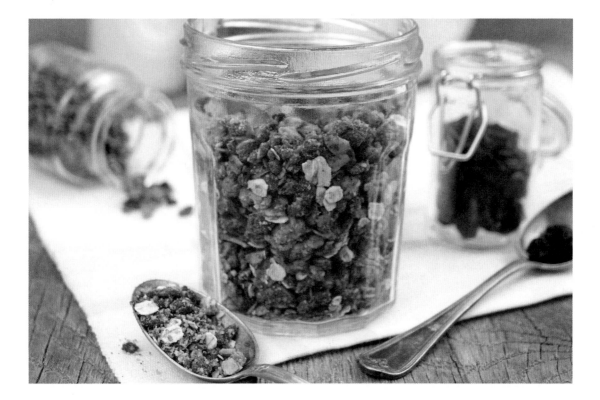

At home	At work	Serves	Kcal	Protein	Carbs	Fat
20 mins	0 min	3	170	4g	11g	12g

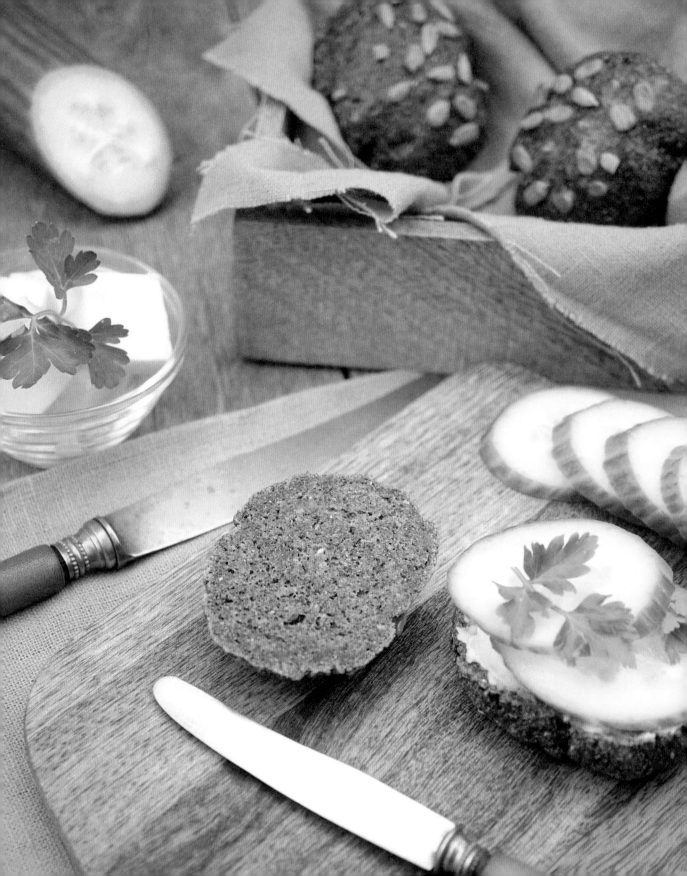

BREADS AND

SPREADS

Blueberry vanilla spread

fruity and delicious

2½oz (75g) blueberries
  (fresh or frozen)
2 tbsp chia seeds
1 tsp vanilla powder
2 tbsp agave syrup

Place the blueberries in a high-sided container and use a hand-held blender to purée them thoroughly (frozen berries can be blended without defrosting). Stir in the chia seeds, vanilla powder, and agave syrup with a spoon. Leave the spread to stand for at least 30 minutes. Transfer to a lidded jar. Store in the refrigerator for up to 1 week.

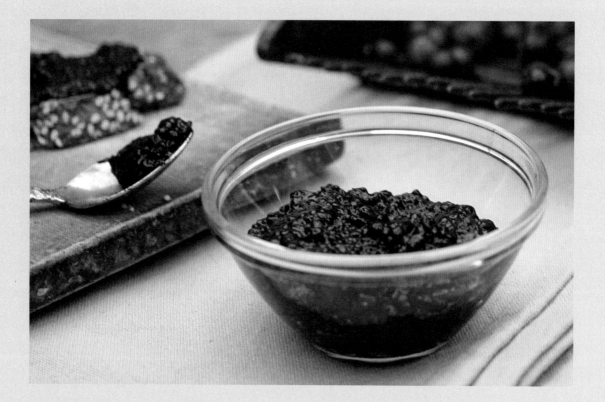

At home	At work	Serves	Kcal	Protein	Carbs	Fat
5 + 30 mins	0 min	5	40	1g	5g	1g

Raspberry chia spread

a taste of summer

2½oz (75g) raspberries
   (fresh or frozen)
2 tbsp chia seeds
1 tbsp agave syrup

Place the raspberries in a high-sided container and use a hand-held blender to purée them thoroughly (frozen berries can be blended without defrosting). Stir in the chia seeds and syrup with a spoon. Leave the spread to stand for at least 30 minutes. Transfer to a lidded jar. Store in the refrigerator for up to 1 week.

OUR TIP—Leave the spread out overnight before using.

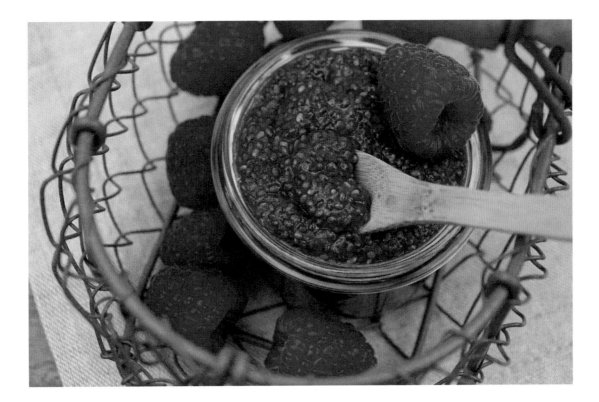

At home	At work	Serves	Kcal	Protein	Carbs	Fat
5 + 30 mins	0 min	5	30	1g	3g	1g

Cashew butter

alternative to butter

3½oz (100g) cashews
1 tbsp sunflower oil

Lightly toast the cashew nuts in a pan without any oil, turning them regularly.

Place the toasted cashews in a high-sided container together with the sunflower oil and use a hand-held blender to purée them as finely as possible.

Transfer the cashew butter to a lidded jar. Can be stored in the refrigerator for at least 4 weeks.

At home	At work	Serves	Kcal	Protein	Carbs	Fat
5 mins	0 min	5	135	3g	6g	10g

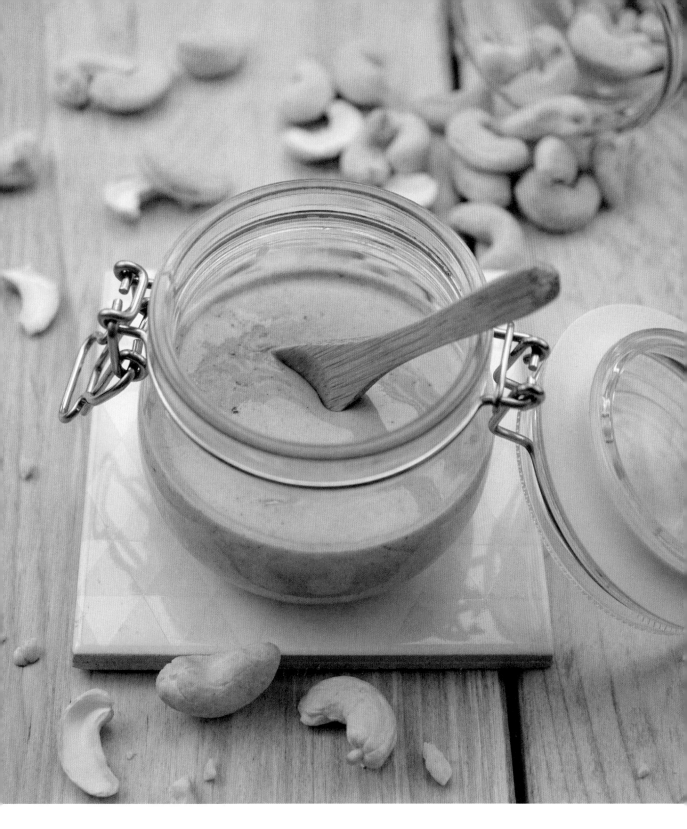

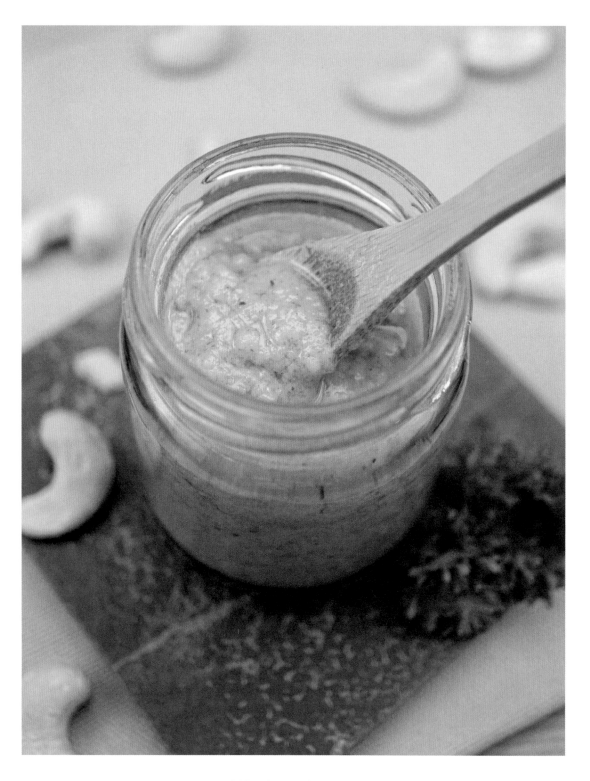

Cashew citrus cream

zesty and aromatic

1¼oz (40g) cashews
salt and freshly ground
   black pepper
1–2 sprigs parsley (curly
   or flat leaf, as desired)
3 mint leaves
2 tbsp olive oil
1 tbsp orange juice
1 tsp lemon juice
1 tsp agave syrup
1 tsp organic lemon zest

Place the cashews in a bowl with 3fl oz (90ml) water and a pinch of salt, and leave to soak for at least 1 hour. Then strain off the water in a sieve, rinse the cashews, and leave to drain.

Transfer the cashews to a high-sided container and add the herbs, followed by the olive oil, orange juice, lemon juice, agave syrup, lemon zest, and a pinch of salt and pepper. Using a hand-held blender, purée the ingredients thoroughly.

Decant the cashew citrus cream into a lidded jar. Can be stored in the refrigerator for several days.

At home	At work	Serves	Kcal	Protein	Carbs	Fat
5 + 60 mins	0 min	5	100	1g	3g	9g

Cucumber radish yogurt

with beet sprouts

3½oz (100g) plain Greek
   yogurt (thick)
3oz (85g) cucumber, peeled
   and cut into cubes
4 radishes, finely chopped
2 sprigs of flat leaf parsley,
   leaves removed and
   finely chopped
salt and freshly ground
   black pepper
1 tbsp beet sprouts

Place the Greek yogurt, cucumber, radishes, and parsley in a bowl, combine, and season with salt and pepper. Transfer the yogurt mixture to a jar. Either add the sprouts directly on top or pack them separately. Put the lid on the jar and store the spread in the refrigerator until ready to serve.

AT WORK—Stir the Greek yogurt thoroughly, then spread it on some low-carb rolls (see p. 77) or similar. If you packed the sprouts separately, scatter them over the yogurt.

At home	At work	Serves	Kcal	Protein	Carbs	Fat
5 mins	1 min	1	122	11g	7g	5g

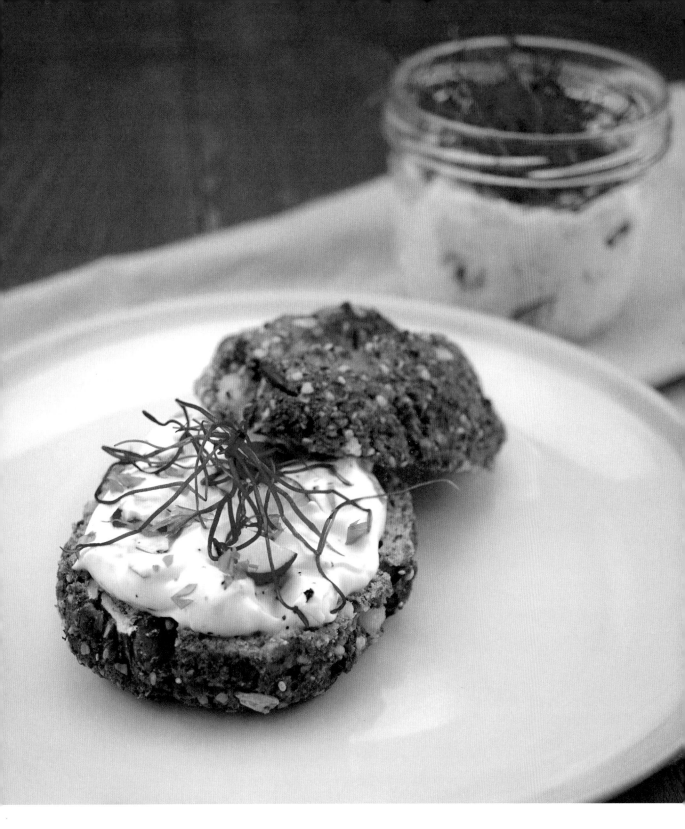

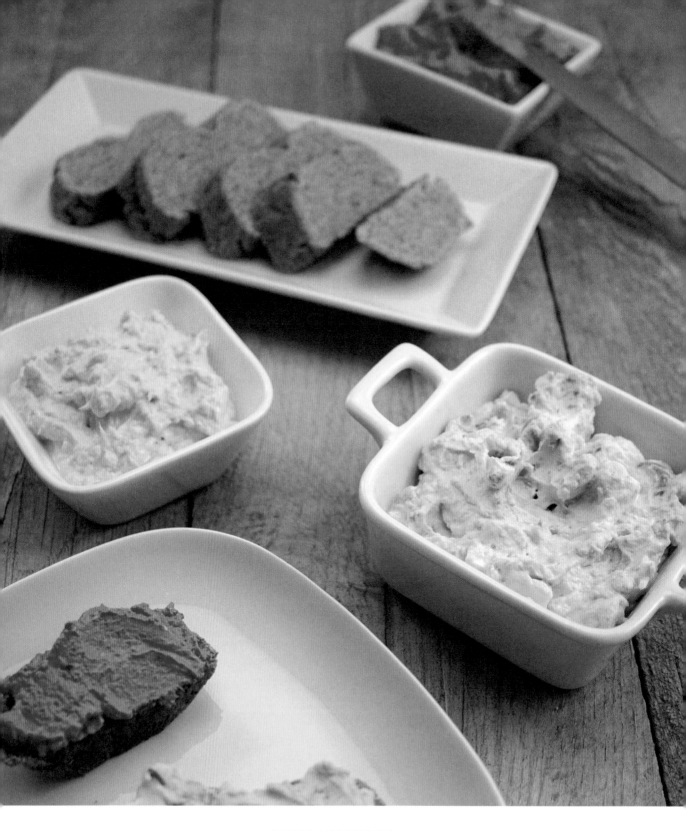

Three kinds of dips

for all your sandwich breaks

BEET DIP

1oz (30g) cooked beets
3oz (85g) full-fat cream cheese
1 splash lemon juice
pinch of low-calorie sweetener,
    such as stevia
salt and freshly ground
    black pepper

Peel and chop the beets, then purée using a hand-held blender. Stir in the cream cheese, lemon juice, and the sweetener. Season the dip to taste.

At home	At work	Serves	Kcal	Protein	Carbs	Fat
5 mins	0 min	4	235	6g	15g	20g

TUNA DIP

1 scant oz (25g) canned tuna
½ shallot, finely chopped
2oz (60g) full-fat cream cheese
1 tsp capers, chopped
1 tsp lemon juice
salt and freshly ground
    black pepper

Drain the tuna and squeeze it out using a paper towel. Place the tuna fish and shallots in a high-sided container and use a hand-held blender to process them to a lumpy consistency. Add the cream cheese, capers, and lemon juice to the tuna purée, and stir until well combined. Season the dip to taste.

At home	At work	Serves	Kcal	Protein	Carbs	Fat
5 mins	0 min	4	200	11g	2g	16g

TOMATO DIP

1oz (30g) sundried tomatoes in oil
2oz (60g) full-fat cream cheese
splash of lime juice
salt and freshly ground
    black pepper

Drain and chop the tomatoes, then place them in a high-sided container and use a hand-held blender to process them to a lumpy consistency. Stir in the cream cheese and lime juice. Season the dip to taste.

At home	At work	Serves	Kcal	Protein	Carbs	Fat
5 mins	0 min	4	220	6g	7g	18g

Goat cheese spread

Mediterranean style

3½fl oz (100ml) olive oil
2 sprigs of rosemary, leaves
   picked and roughly chopped
sprig of thyme, leaves picked
   and roughly chopped
1 tsp dried basil
5 sundried tomatoes in oil,
   finely chopped
1¼oz (40g) goat cheese,
   sliced into two discs

Put the olive oil into a jar with the rosemary, thyme, basil, and tomatoes, then add the goat cheese discs.

Place the lid on the jar and store in the refrigerator until ready to serve. The cheeses will keep for up to approximately 4 weeks in the refrigerator, provided they are always well covered in oil.

OUR TIP—Ideally leave the goat cheese to infuse overnight.

At home	At work	Serves	Kcal	Protein	Carbs	Fat
5 mins	0 min	2	140	5g	4g	11g

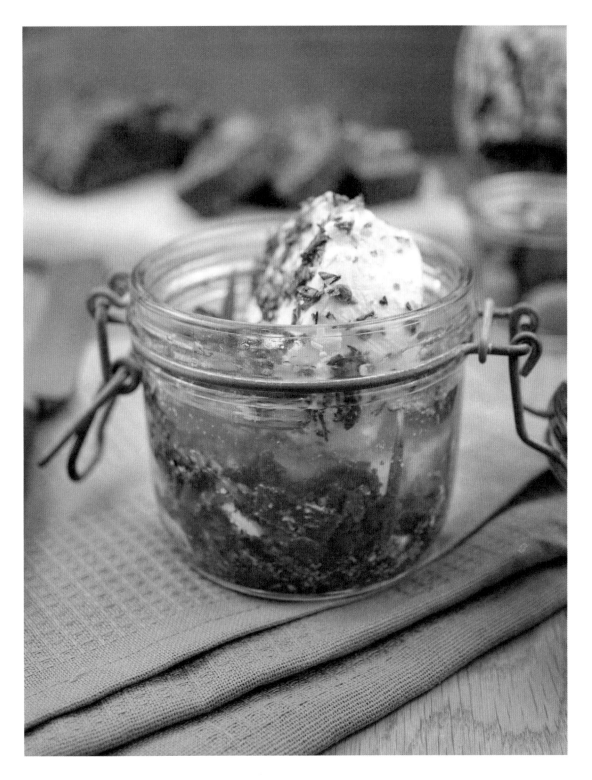

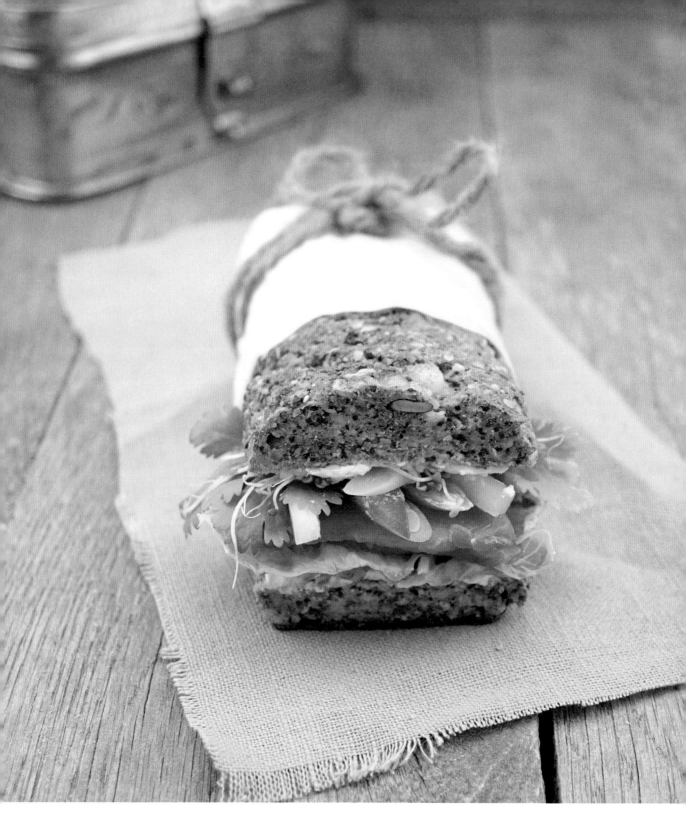

Cottage baguette

wholesome and vital

1oz (30g) ground almonds
1 scant oz (25g) ground
  hazelnuts
1oz (30g) psyllium husks
¼oz (10g) coconut flour
¼oz (10g) cream of tartar
3 eggs
4½oz (125g) cottage cheese
1 tbsp cider vinegar
½ tsp salt
pinch of ground coriander
1oz (30g) shelled hemp seeds
1oz (30g) chia seeds
½oz (15g) sunflower seeds
¼oz (10g) pumpkin seeds

Preheat the oven to 400°F (200°C). Line a baking sheet with parchment paper.

Combine the almonds, hazelnuts, psyllium husks, coconut flour, and cream of tartar in a bowl. Whisk the eggs in a separate bowl and stir in the cottage cheese, cider vinegar, salt, and coriander. Add the nut and flour mixture to the egg mixture and combine everything thoroughly.

Add the hemp, chia, sunflower, and pumpkin seeds to the dough mixture and stir them in. Lay the dough out lengthwise on the parchment paper and shape it into a baguette.

Cut the surface of the dough several times with a knife. Bake the baguette in the center of the oven for 30–40 minutes, until crisp and golden brown. Remove from the sheet and leave to cool on a wire rack. Pack up a portion of the baguette in a container to take with you, leaving it plain or adding a topping, as desired.

OUR TIP—You can instead shape four delicious low-carb cottage rolls from this dough. Just shorten the cooking time to 25–30 minutes.

At home	At work	Serves	Kcal	Protein	Carbs	Fat
10 + 40 mins	0 min	4	305	18g	8g	20g

"Oopsies"

protein buns

3 eggs
3½oz (100g) full-fat
 cream cheese
salt

Preheat the oven to 400°F (200°C). Line 2 baking sheets with parchment paper.

Separate the egg whites from the yolks. Beat the whites in a bowl using a hand-held whisk until they are stiff. In a separate bowl, stir together the cream cheese and egg yolks and season the mixture with a little salt. Fold the beaten egg whites carefully into this mixture using a whisk or spatula.

Using a ladle, immediately scoop 4 dollops of the dough mixture onto each of the baking sheets—making sure the blobs of dough aren't too close, because otherwise the oopsies will merge together.

Bake the oopsies on the lower and central shelf of the oven for 15–20 minutes. Remove from the sheet and leave to cool on a wire rack. Pack them up in a container to take with you, leaving them plain or adding a topping, as desired.

OUR TIP—Oopsies can be filled with whatever topping you like; they also work well as burger buns.

At home	At work	Serves	Kcal	Protein	Carbs	Fat
10 + 20 mins	0 min	8	65	3g	1g	5g

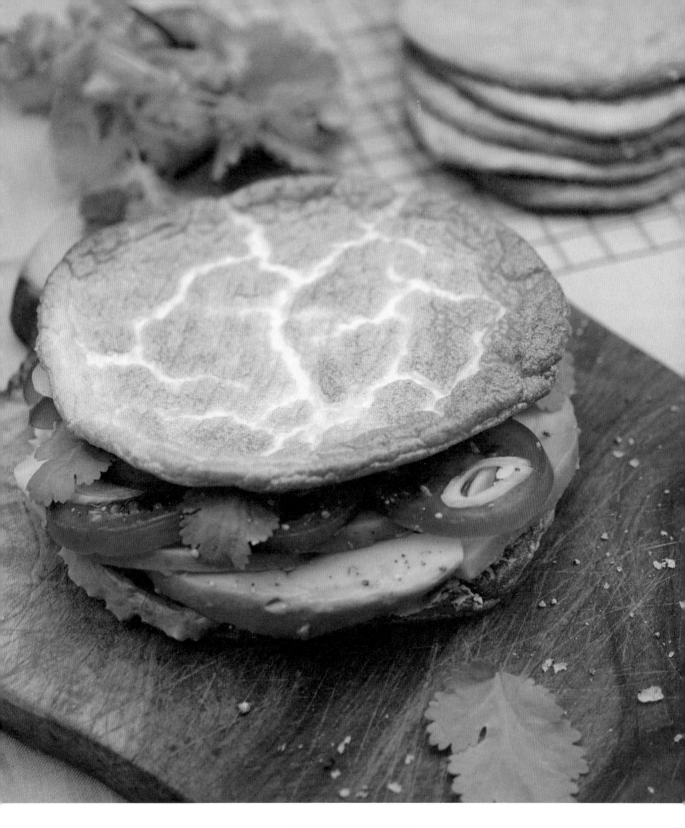

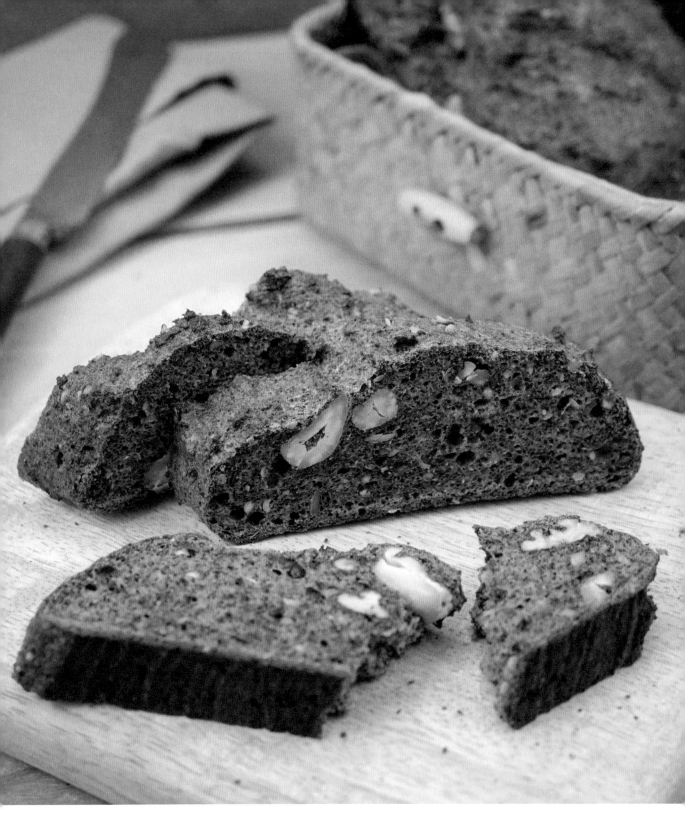

Nut bread
power loaf

---

4 eggs
6oz (175g) plain Greek yogurt (thick)
1 scant oz (25g) cashews
1 scant oz (25g) pecans
¼oz (10g) psyllium husks
½ tsp ground coriander
1 tsp salt
1¾oz (50g) hemp flour
1oz (30g) linseed flour
¼oz (10g) shelled hemp seeds
¼oz (10g) linseeds

Preheat the oven to 350°F (180°C). Line a baking sheet with parchment paper.

Separate the egg whites from the yolks. Beat the egg whites in a bowl using a hand-held whisk until they are stiff. In a separate bowl, stir together the egg yolks and the Greek yogurt.

Roughly chop the cashews and pecans. Mix together the psyllium husks, coriander, salt, hemp and linseed flours, hemp seeds, and linseeds. Stir this mixture into the yogurt mix. Add the cashews and pecans, then carefully fold in the beaten egg whites. Finally, knead everything together to form a dough.

Allow the dough to rest for around 5 minutes, then shape it into a loaf on the parchment paper. Use a knife to make incisions in the top of the loaf, then bake in the center of the oven for 50–60 minutes. Remove the bread from the sheet and leave to cool on a wire rack. Store in a container.

OUR TIP—A practical option for packed lunches is to make two smaller loaves from this dough. The baking time should then be shortened to 35–45 minutes.

At home	At work	Serves	Kcal	Protein	Carbs	Fat
15 + 60 mins	0 min	8	150	10g	3g	9g

Spelt and hemp bread

with sunflower seeds

7g dry yeast (or
  ½ cube fresh yeast)
1 tbsp agave syrup
1 tbsp salt
9oz (250g) whole meal
  spelt flour
8oz (225g) spelt flour with
  a high gluten content
1 scant oz (25g) linseed flour
3 tbsp sunflower seeds
2 tbsp linseeds
2 tbsp shelled hemp seeds
1 tbsp chia seeds

Dissolve the yeast in about 3½ tablespoons of lukewarm water and add the agave syrup. In a large bowl, combine the salt with all the different types of flour, sunflower seeds, linseeds, hemp seeds, and chia seeds.

Gradually add 9–10fl oz (250–300ml) lukewarm water to the yeast liquid, then knead everything together thoroughly for 5–10 minutes, until you have a stretchy dough. If the dough remains too sticky, knead in a bit of additional flour. Leave the dough covered in a warm place for around 1 hour to proof, until it has roughly doubled in size.

Preheat the oven to 425°F (220°C). Line a loaf pan with parchment paper. Knead the bread dough thoroughly once more, shape it into a loaf, and place it in the pan. Bake the bread in the center of the oven for around 15 minutes, then lower the oven temperature to 325°F (160°C) and continue to bake the bread for an additional 15–20 minutes, until done.

Remove from the oven and leave the bread to cool in the pan for about 10 minutes, then release it from the pan and allow to cool down completely on a wire rack. Store in a container.

At home	At work	Serves	Kcal	Protein	Carbs	Fat
15 + 95 mins	0 min	16	130	6g	21g	2g

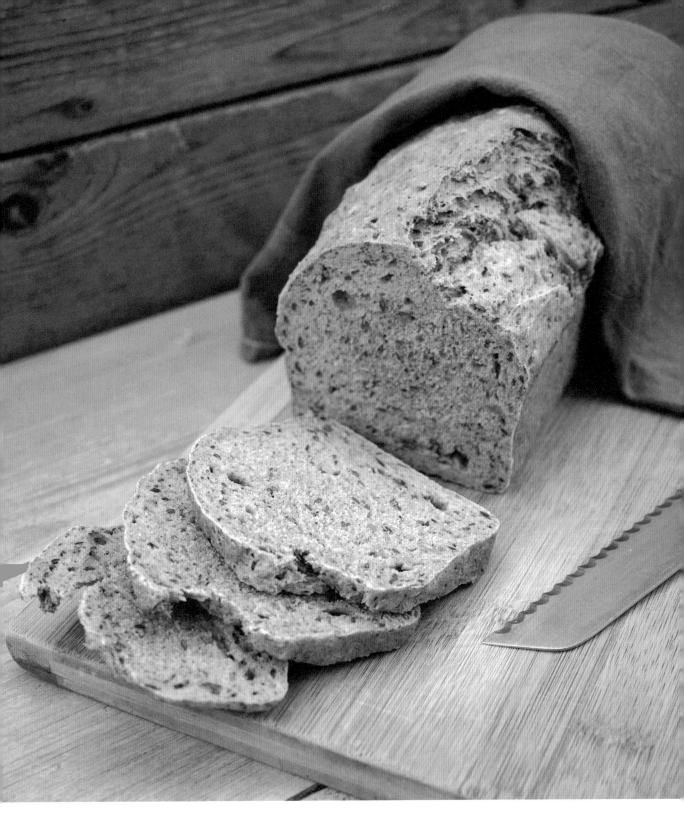

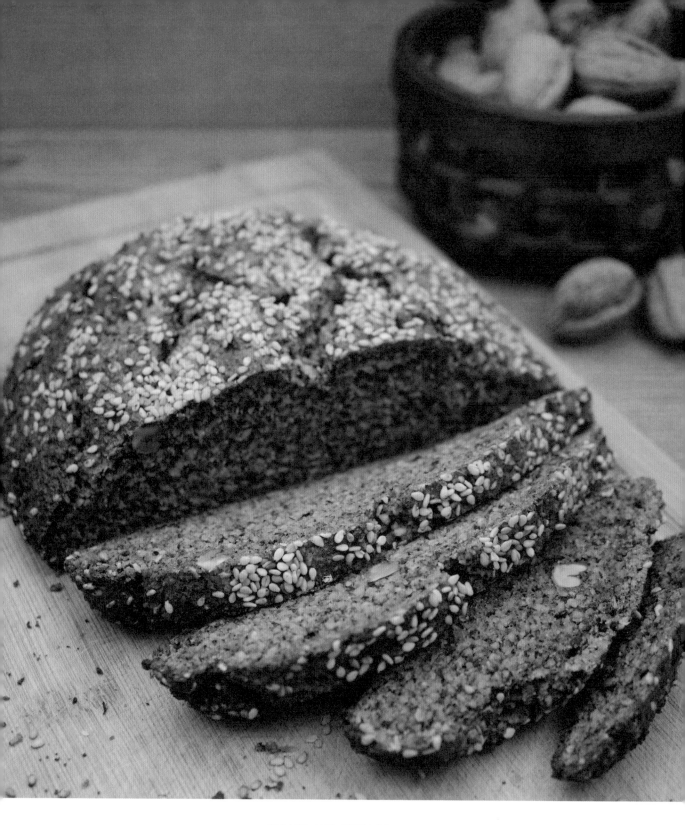

Walnut bread

with crunchy nuts

6 whole walnuts
1oz (30g) soft butter
2 eggs
3 tbsp yogurt
about 1 tsp agave syrup
pinch of salt
2 tbsp ground walnuts
7oz (200g) ground almonds
½ tsp baking soda
2 tbsp white sesame seeds

Preheat the oven to 400°F (200°C). Line a baking sheet with parchment paper.

Crack open the 6 walnuts, remove the kernels from their shells, and chop roughly. Beat the butter in a bowl using a hand-held whisk until light and fluffy, then add the eggs and mix everything well. Stir the yogurt, agave syrup, and salt into the butter and egg mixture.

In a separate bowl, combine the ground walnuts, almonds, and baking soda. Add this nut mixture to the egg mixture and stir together to form a dough. Finally, mix in the chopped walnuts.

Shape or press the dough to create a round loaf on the parchment paper. Scatter the loaf with sesame seeds and press these in slightly. Bake the walnut bread in the center of the oven for 30 minutes, then lower the temperature to 350°F (180°C) and cook the bread for an additional 10–15 minutes, until done.

Remove the bread from the sheet and leave to cool on a wire rack. Store in a container.

At home	At work	Serves	Kcal	Protein	Carbs	Fat
15 + 45 mins	0 min	10	200	8g	2g	17g

Buttermilk rolls

lovingly homemade

9oz (250g) buttermilk
½ cube of yeast (scant 1oz/25g)
12oz (350g) spelt flour with a
    high gluten content
1 tsp honey or a bit of
    low-calorie sweetener
    such as stevia
1 tsp salt

In a saucepan, heat the buttermilk until lukewarm, then dissolve the yeast into it. Add the flour, honey, and salt, and knead together to form a dough. Cover the dough and leave to proof in a warm place for around 30 minutes. Knead again and use some flour to help you shape 6 rolls from the mixture. Line a baking sheet with parchment paper. Leave the rolls to proof on the sheet for 15 minutes. Preheat the oven to 425°F (220°C). Bake the rolls in the center of the oven for 15–20 minutes. Remove and leave to cool, then pack them in a container.

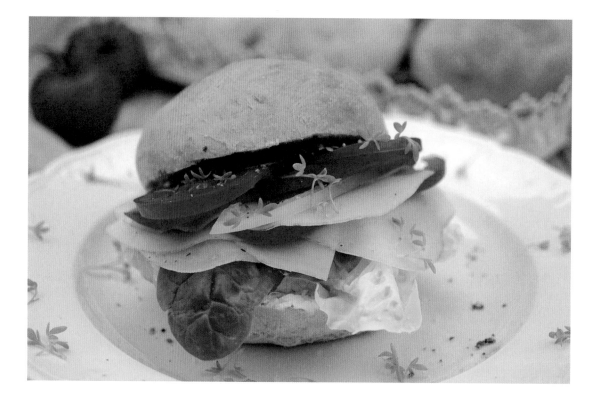

At home	At work	Serves	Kcal	Protein	Carbs	Fat
25 + 65 mins	0 min	6	220	9g	41g	1g

Low-carb rolls
with sunflower seeds

1¾oz (50g) linseed flour
½oz (15g) coconut flour
¼oz (10g) ground walnuts
½oz (15g) psyllium husks
1 tsp cream of tartar
1 tsp salt
1 tsp dried oregano
1oz (30g) sunflower seeds
⅛oz (5g) chia seeds
1 egg white

In a large bowl, combine all the ingredients except the egg white. Stir in 4½fl oz (130ml) boiling water with a fork, then knead everything by hand. Beat the egg white until stiff, add to the mixture, and knead everything together until you have a consistent dough. Line a baking sheet with parchment paper. Shape the dough into 3 rolls; leave these to rest on the baking sheet for 10 minutes. Preheat the oven to 350°F (180°C). Bake the rolls in the center of the oven for around 30 minutes. Remove, allow to cool, then pack them up in a container to take with you.

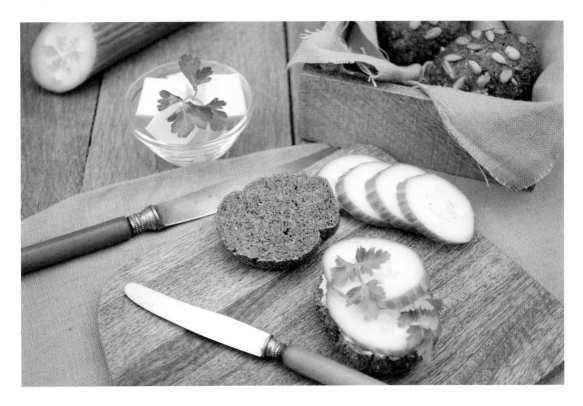

At home	At work	Serves	Kcal	Protein	Carbs	Fat
30 + 30 mins	0 min	3	180	11g	6g	8g

Fitness baguette

with a delicate hint of fennel, anise, and caraway

1 bag fennel, anise, and
  caraway tea
1oz (30g) linseed flour
1oz (30g) ground almonds
1¼oz (40g) coconut flour
½oz (15g) psyllium husk powder
½ tsp salt
½oz (15g) cream of tartar
2 eggs
5 ½oz (150g) plain Greek
  yogurt (thick)
1 tsp cider vinegar

Place the tea bag in a mug, pour boiling hot water over it, and leave to steep for 10 minutes.

In a bowl, combine the linseed flour, almonds, coconut flour, and psyllium husks, then stir in the salt and cream of tartar. In a separate bowl, mix together the eggs, yogurt, and vinegar. Add 1½ tablespoons of hot tea and the egg-yogurt mix to the dry ingredients and knead everything together to form a dough.

Line a baking sheet with parchment paper. Shape the dough into a loaf and place this on the parchment paper, making several diagonal incisions in the surface with a knife. Leave the dough to proof for 30 minutes.

Meanwhile, preheat the oven to 400°F (200°C). Bake the bread in the center of the oven for 40–50 minutes, until golden brown. Remove from the sheet and leave to cool on a wire rack. Store the baguette in a container until ready to use.

At home	At work	Serves	Kcal	Protein	Carbs	Fat
15 + 80 mins	0 min	4	180	14g	8g	8g

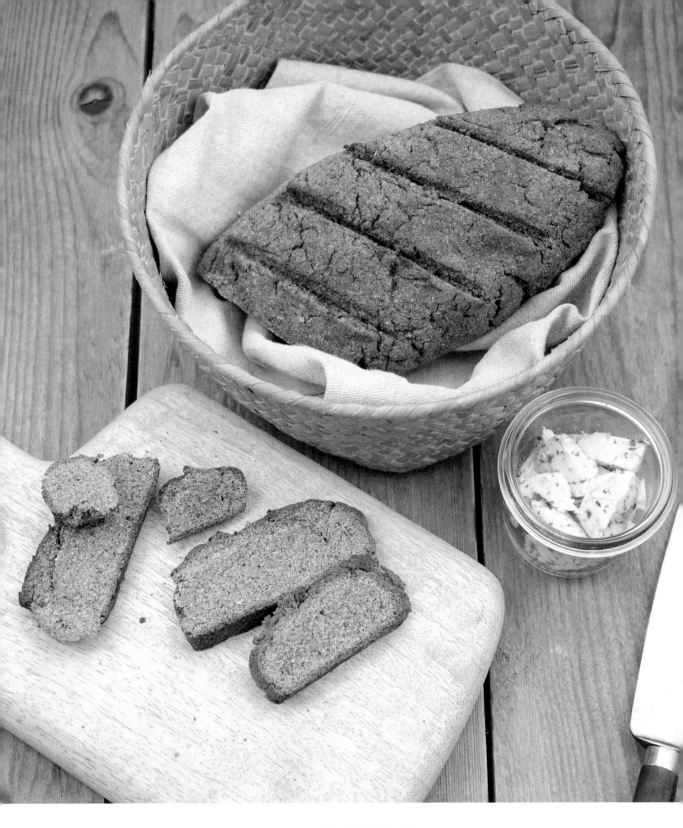

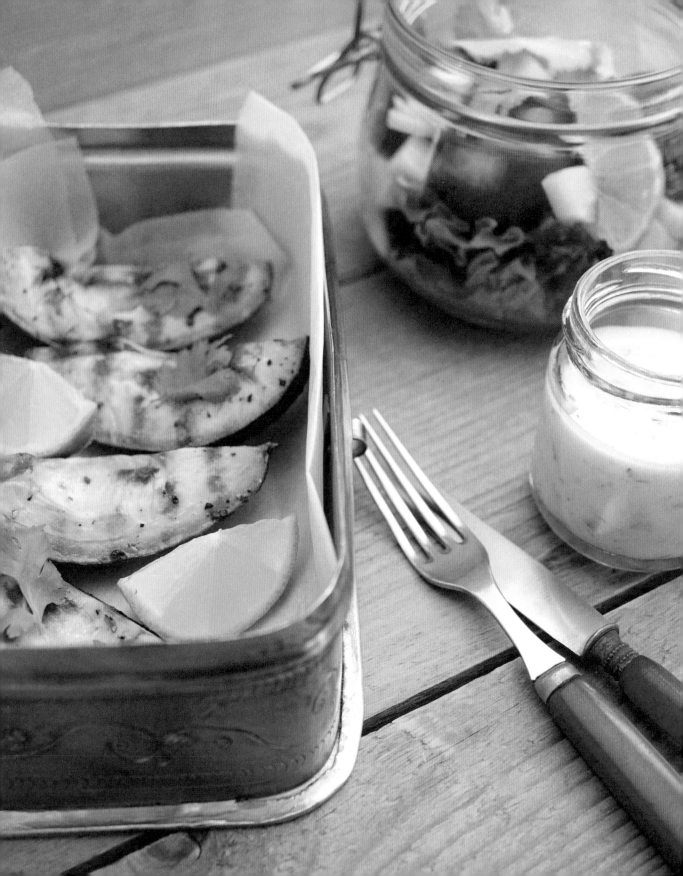

VEGETARIAN

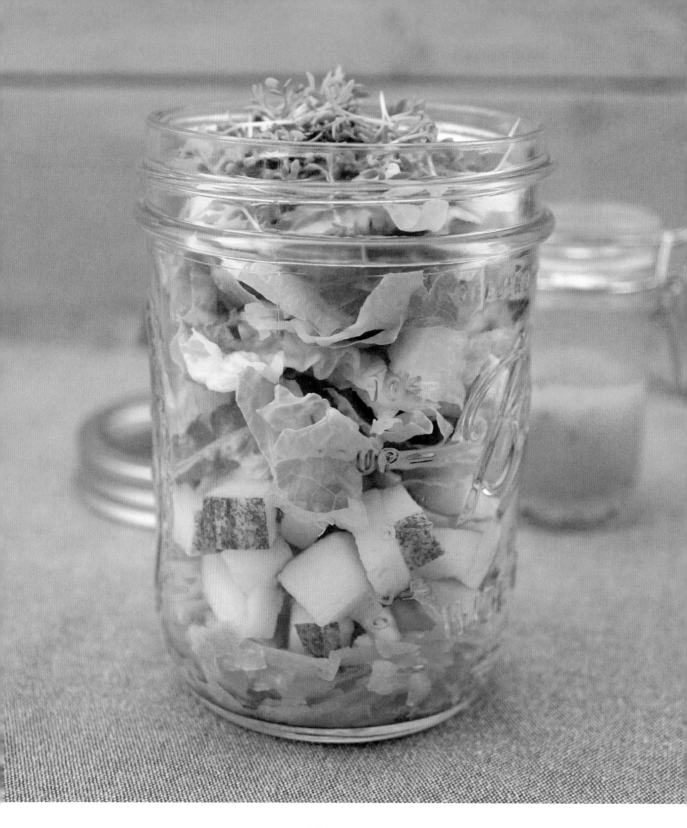

VEGETARIAN

Apple and carrot salad
with watercress

FOR THE SALAD
1 carrot, finely grated
2 tsp lemon juice
1 tsp olive oil
1 small apple, cored and cut
    into bite-sized cubes
½ romaine lettuce, roughly
    chopped
1 tbsp watercress leaves

FOR THE DRESSING
3 tbsp olive oil
2 tbsp lemon juice
1 tbsp orange juice
1 tsp cress leaves
salt and freshly ground
    black pepper

Drizzle the carrot with about 1 tsp lemon juice and the olive oil. Drizzle the diced apple with the remaining lemon juice.

Layer the grated carrot, apple, and lettuce in a tall jar and finish off with the watercress leaves. Close the jar.

To make the dressing, put all the ingredients into a small jar. Seal the jar and shake vigorously so the ingredients combine to form a homogenous dressing. Store the salad and dressing in the refrigerator until ready to serve.

AT WORK—Shake the dressing again in the closed jar, then add to the salad.

At home	At work	Serves	Kcal	Protein	Carbs	Fat
10 mins	1 min	1	380	2g	17g	32g

Carrot and cucumber noodles
with lime dressing

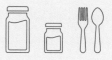

FOR THE SALAD
1 carrot
½ cucumber, peeled
1 tbsp white sesame seeds
½ romaine lettuce, cut into
   thin strips
1 scallion, root discarded,
   white part thinly sliced
¼ red chili, seeded and
   thinly sliced
salt and freshly ground
   black pepper

FOR THE DRESSING
juice of ½ lime
2 ½ tbsp olive oil
1 tbsp sesame oil
1 tsp agave syrup
½ tsp salt

Use a spiralizer to cut the carrot and cucumber into long vegetable noodles. Toast the sesame seeds in a dry pan until they release their aroma.

Combine all the prepared salad ingredients carefully in a salad bowl. Season the salad with salt and pepper, transfer to a tall jar, and close.

For the dressing, place all the ingredients in a bowl and mix thoroughly. Pour the dressing into a small jar and close. Store the salad and dressing in the refrigerator until ready to serve.

AT WORK—Add the dressing to the salad, close the jar, and shake. Eat the salad straight from the jar or tip it out onto a plate.

At home	At work	Serves	Kcal	Protein	Carbs	Fat
10 mins	1 min	1	169	4g	15g	11g

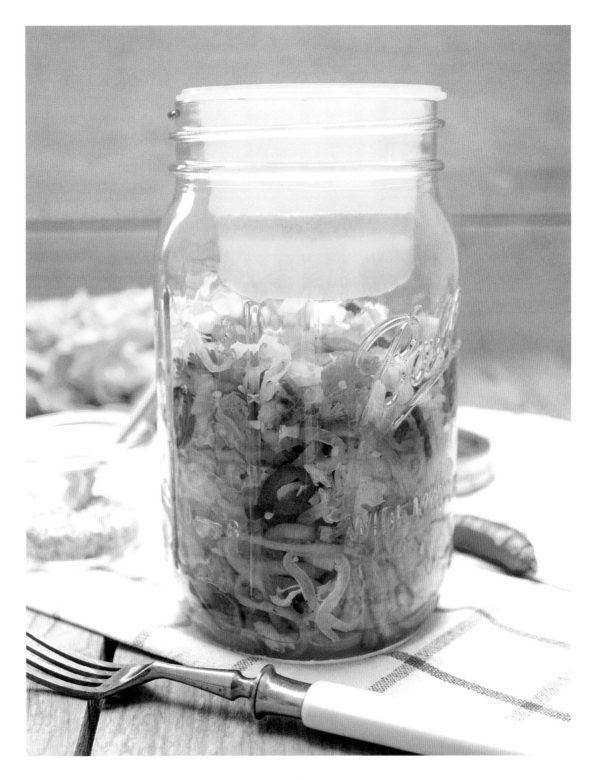

VEGETARIAN

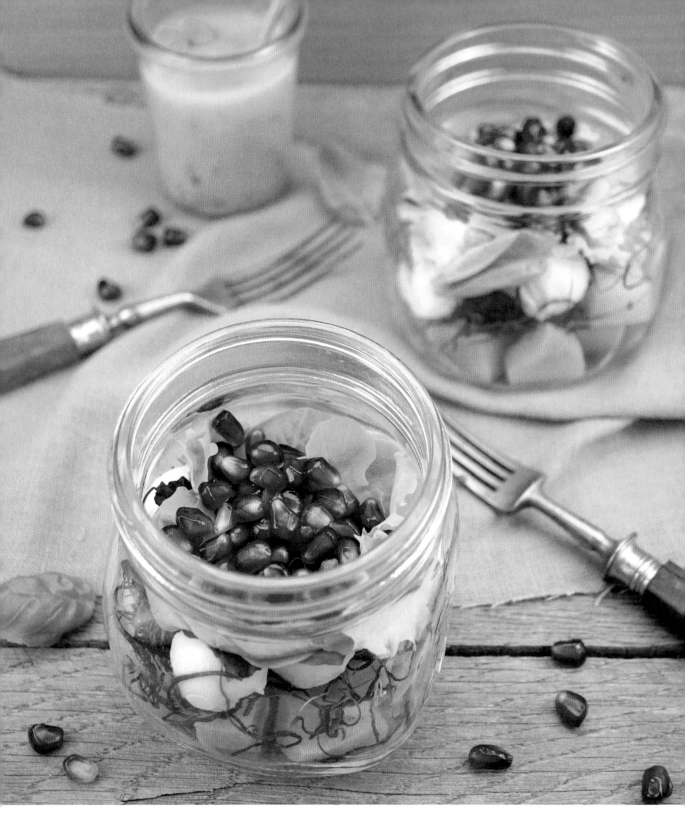

VEGETARIAN

Squash salad

with a basil and squash dressing

10oz (300g) butternut squash,
   peeled, seeds removed, and
   cut into small cubes
slice of ginger, peeled
2 sprigs of basil leaves
1 tsp peanut oil
salt and freshly ground
   black pepper
2 tbsp beet sprouts
10 mini mozzarella balls
2–3 round lettuce leaves,
   roughly chopped
2 tbsp pomegranate seeds

Preheat the oven to 350°F (180°C). Line a baking sheet with parchment paper. Spread the squash over the parchment paper and roast in the center of the oven for around 15 minutes, until soft but not mushy. Remove the squash from the oven and leave to cool.

To make the dressing, put around 2oz (60g) of the cooked squash into a blender beaker. Add the ginger, basil, peanut oil, and 2½fl oz (75ml) water to the squash and use a hand-held blender to process thoroughly. Season the dressing with salt and pepper to taste and pour into a small jar. Close the jar and keep the dressing in the refrigerator until ready to use.

To make the salad, divide the remaining squash between 2 jars. Rinse the sprouts briefly in cold water in a strainer, drain thoroughly, then add to the squash. Place the mozzarella balls on top. Add the lettuce leaves on top of the mozzarella balls and finish off with the pomegranate seeds. Close the jars and store the salad in the refrigerator until ready to serve.

AT WORK—Tip the salad out onto a plate and drizzle the dressing over it using a spoon. Or pour the dressing over the salad in the jar and eat it straight from the container.

At home	At work	Serves	Kcal	Protein	Carbs	Fat
30 mins	1 min	2	185	8g	18g	9g

Multicolored salad

with quinoa

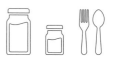

FOR THE SALAD

1 tsp pine nuts
1oz (30g) quinoa
1 tsp orange juice
salt and freshly ground
    black pepper
7 cherry tomatoes, halved
2oz (60g) orange bell pepper,
    seeded and finely chopped
1¼oz (40g) yellow bell pepper,
    seeded and finely chopped
1 red cabbage leaf, about
    ¾oz (20g), thinly sliced
1 round lettuce leaf, finely
    chopped

FOR THE DRESSING

2 tbsp orange juice
1 tbsp lemon juice
1–2 tsp agave syrup (to taste)

Toast the pine nuts in a dry pan until golden brown, remove from the pan, and leave to cool.

Wash the quinoa thoroughly in a strainer under running water. Transfer the quinoa to a pan, cover with water, and simmer uncovered for 8–10 minutes, until cooked. Drain the water, stir the orange juice into the quinoa, and leave to soak briefly. Season the orange quinoa with salt and pepper to taste and leave to cool.

To make the dressing, stir together the orange and lemon juices. Sweeten the dressing to taste with some agave syrup, then pour into a small jar and seal. Store the dressing in the refrigerator until ready to use.

Transfer the quinoa to a jar, then arrange layers of tomatoes, bell pepper pieces, cabbage, and lettuce one after the other, finishing off with a scattering of pine nuts. Close the jar and keep the salad in the refrigerator until you are ready to serve.

AT WORK—Add the dressing to the salad and eat straight from the jar, or serve on a plate.

At home	At work	Serves	Kcal	Protein	Carbs	Fat
15 mins	1 min	1	170	5g	23g	5g

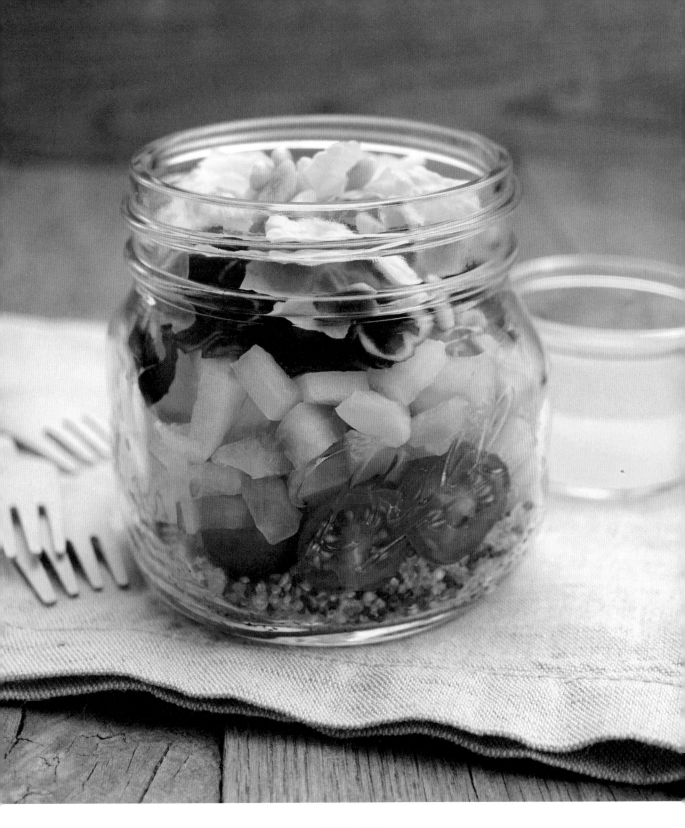

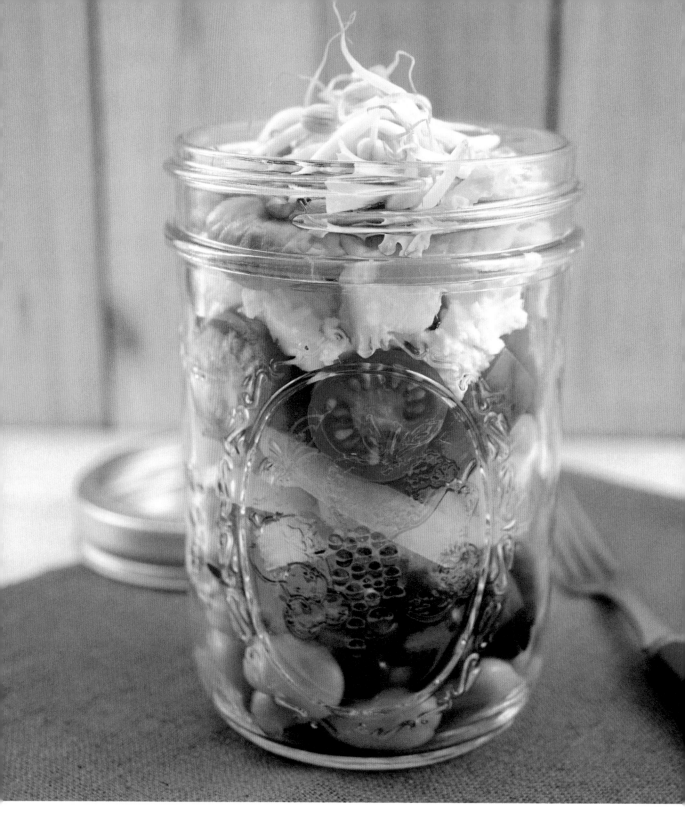

VEGETARIAN

Bell pepper and bean salad
with feta

1¾oz (50g) canned navy
   or cannellini beans
1¾oz (50g) canned kidney
   beans
small piece of orange bell
   pepper, about 1 scant oz
   (25g), seeded and sliced
   into strips
small piece of red bell pepper,
   about 1 scant oz (25g),
   seeded and sliced
   into strips
2 yellow cherry tomatoes,
   halved
1 red cherry tomato, halved
1oz (30g) feta
handful of mixed lettuce leaves,
   roughly chopped
1 tbsp bean sprouts
salt and freshly ground black
   pepper (in lidded dispensers)

Rinse the navy or cannellini beans and the kidney beans thoroughly in a strainer under running water and leave to drain. Transfer all the beans to a jar.

Layer the bell pepper strips on top of the beans. Add the tomatoes to the jar. Crumble the feta with your fingers and scatter over the tomatoes, then add the lettuce to the jar.

Blanch the bean sprouts in boiling water for about 5 seconds, rinse under cold water in a strainer, and leave to drain. Scatter the bean sprouts over the salad. Close the jar and store the salad in the refrigerator until ready to serve.

AT WORK—Pour the salad out onto a plate and season with salt and pepper. Alternatively, eat the salad straight from the jar.

At home	At work	Serves	Kcal	Protein	Carbs	Fat
10 mins	1 min	1	190	14g	14g	7g

Tomato salad with cottage cheese
and basil

7oz (200g) cottage cheese
salt and freshly ground
　　black pepper
zest and juice of 1 organic
　　lemon
2 sprigs of basil leaves
1 tsp olive oil
5 red cherry tomatoes, halved
5 yellow cherry tomatoes,
　　halved
3 radishes, thinly sliced

Season the cottage cheese with salt and pepper and stir in the lemon zest.

Using a mortar and pestle, grind the basil leaves with the olive oil, pepper, and 1–2 tablespoons of lemon juice to create the dressing. Transfer the dressing to a bowl and toss the tomatoes and radishes into it.

Pack up the cottage cheese and tomato salad in 2 separate containers and close them. Store both in the refrigerator until ready to serve.

AT WORK—Add the tomato salad to the cottage cheese and eat straight from the container. Or arrange the cheese and salad together on a plate.

At home	At work	Serves	Kcal	Protein	Carbs	Fat
10 mins	1 min	1	270	26g	9g	14g

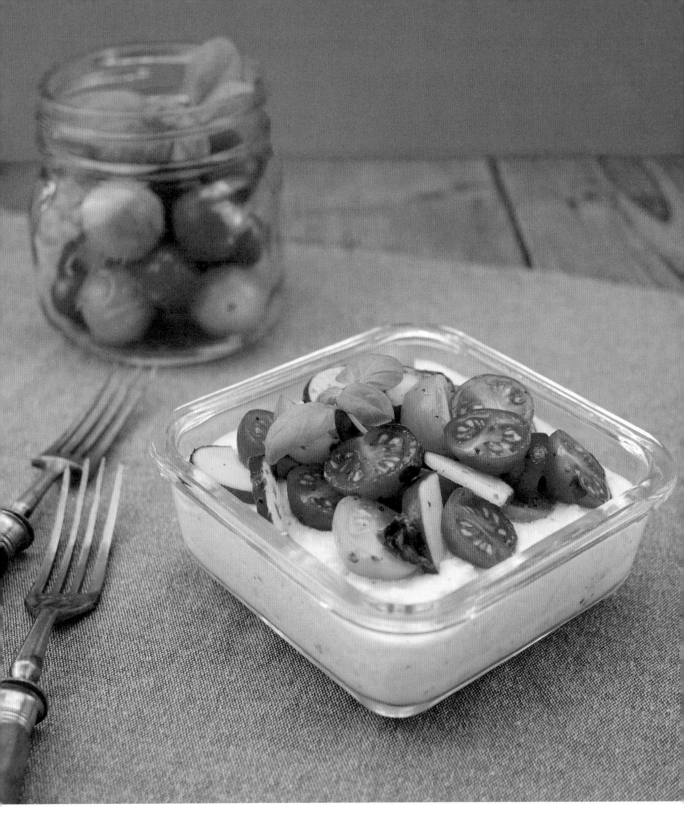

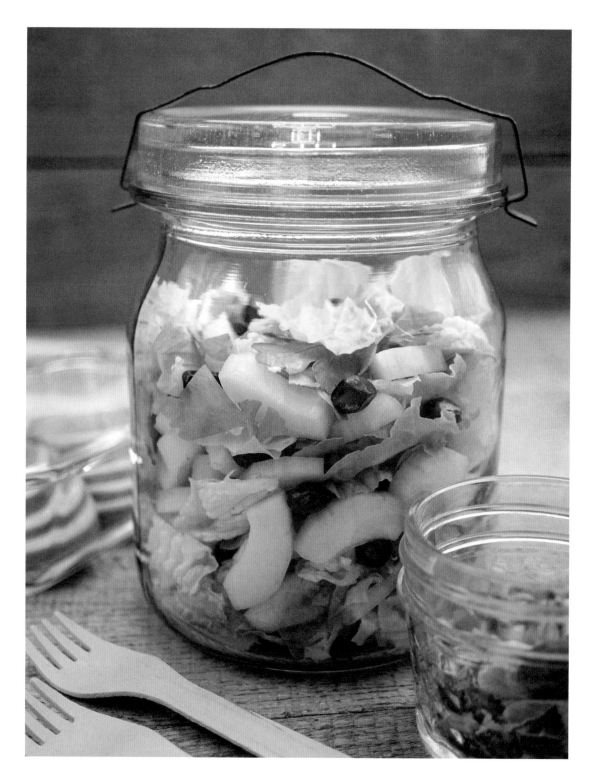

VEGETARIAN

Cucumber power
with avocado

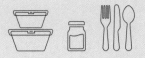

½ cucumber, sliced lengthwise, seeds removed, and chopped into small pieces
2 handfuls of green salad, roughly chopped
1–2 sprigs of cilantro leaves
1 tbsp pomegranate seeds
1 avocado, pitted, flesh removed, and sliced
juice of ½ lime
2 tbsp mixed nuts
1 tbsp white sesame seeds
salt and freshly ground pepper (in lidded dispensers)

Place the cucumber, salad, and cilantro in a container. Add the pomegranate seeds.

Drizzle the avocado slices with lime juice to prevent them from going brown. Pack the avocado slices into a separate container. Put the mixed nuts and sesame seeds into another container. Close all your containers and store the salad mixture and the avocado in the refrigerator until ready to serve.

AT WORK—Arrange your cucumber power salad on 2 plates and season with salt and pepper. Add the avocado and the nut mixture. The salad can be drizzled with some lime juice or olive oil or with a salad dressing (for example, from the apple and carrot salad, see p. 83, or from the carrot and cucumber noodles, see p. 84).

At home	At work	Serves	Kcal	Protein	Carbs	Fat
10 mins	2 mins	2	330	6g	5g	32g

Kimchi

spicy Korean Chinese cabbage

10oz (300g) Chinese cabbage, tough stems removed and leaves roughly chopped
½ carrot, cut into matchsticks
½ scallion, root discarded, white part thinly sliced
2 tbsp salt
2 garlic cloves, crushed
2 tbsp soy sauce
2 tbsp chili flakes

Place the cabbage, carrot, and scallion in a bowl, sprinkle with the salt, and leave to steep for 30 minutes. Transfer the vegetables to a strainer, then rinse them off thoroughly under cold water and leave to drain. Use your hands to squeeze any excess water from the vegetables and transfer to a large bowl.

Put the garlic in a small bowl. Add the soy sauce and chili flakes and stir. Add this mixture to the cabbage and combine everything thoroughly with your hands, working the ingredients for several minutes.

Either eat the kimchi immediately, or transfer it to a sterile, dry jar with a sealed lid, filling the jar only three-quarters full, and leave it to mature in the refrigerator. The kimchi will gradually collapse down in the jar. The longer the kimchi is left to infuse in the refrigerator, the more aromatic its flavor becomes. Kimchi can be kept refrigerated for at least 2 weeks, and often much longer.

OUR TIP—If you feel like experimenting with kimchi a bit, add a sweet element, perhaps in the form of some puréed apple or pear.

At home	At work	Serves	Kcal	Protein	Carbs	Fat
45 mins	0 min	4	40	2g	5g	1g

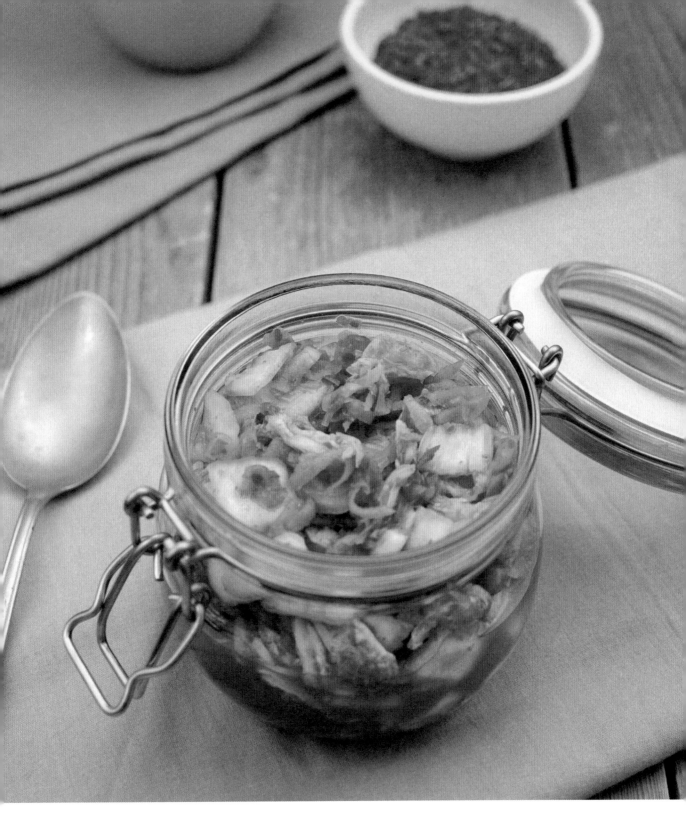

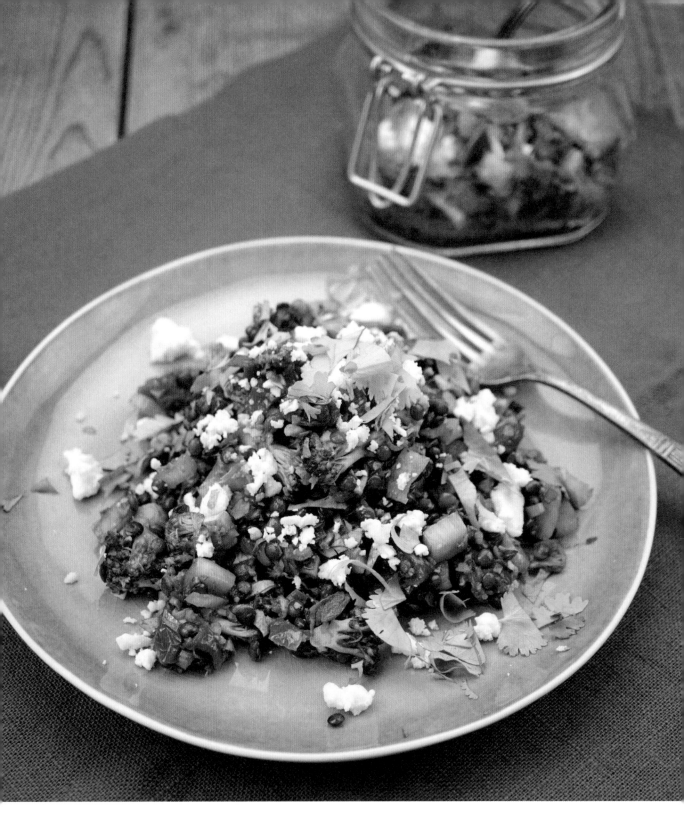

Beluga lentil salad
with feta

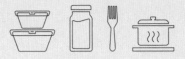

1¾oz (50g) beluga lentils
1 tbsp coconut oil
1 shallot, finely diced
2 tsp tomato purée
1 tbsp cider vinegar
2oz (60g) broccoli florets
2oz (60g) fennel, thinly sliced
1 scallion, root discarded and
    white part finely sliced
grated zest of 1 organic lemon
3 tbsp soy sauce
pinch of ground star anise
pinch of ground cumin
salt and freshly ground
    black pepper
1 tsp goji berries
1 pecan nut
1 small sun-dried tomato
1oz (30g) feta
2 sprigs of cilantro

Cover the beluga lentils with water in a bowl and leave to soak for 12 hours, ideally overnight. Drain the lentils in a strainer and rinse with water.

Heat the coconut oil in a small pan and sauté the shallot. Add the lentils plus the tomato purée and stir everything together. Deglaze with the cider vinegar and 3½ tablespoons of water and leave to simmer for 15 minutes. Add the broccoli, fennel, and scallion and top up with 2–3½fl oz (60–100ml) water. Simmer for 10 more minutes, until the lentils are just cooked.

Stir the lemon zest, soy sauce, star anise, cumin, and some salt and pepper into the lentils. Finely chop the goji berries, pecans, and sun-dried tomato and stir these in, too. Remove the pan from the heat and leave the lentil salad to cool down. Transfer to a jar and seal. Pack the feta and cilantro in a separate container and store this in the refrigerator with the salad until ready to serve.

AT WORK—If desired, heat the salad in a pan. Crumble the feta over the salad with your fingers. Wash and dab the cilantro dry, pluck off the leaves, chop coarsely, and add to the salad.

At home	At work	Serves	Kcal	Protein	Carbs	Fat
20 mins + 12 hrs	5 mins	2	225	12g	17g	11g

Red lentil salad
with harissa dressing

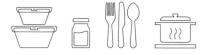

FOR THE SALAD
1 tbsp olive oil
1 shallot, diced
2¼oz (70g) red lentils
½–¾in (1–2cm) piece of
    ginger, grated
1 garlic clove, diced
7fl oz (200ml) vegetable stock
1½oz (45g) zucchini, cut into cubes
1¾oz (50g) red bell pepper,
    seeded and cut into cubes
sprig of rosemary leaves,
    finely chopped
salt and freshly ground
    black pepper
1½oz (45g) spinach leaves,
    roughly chopped

FOR THE DRESSING
3 tbsp yogurt
½ tsp harissa paste
1 tsp lemon juice

FOR THE TOPPING
sprig of mint
sprig of flat-leaf parsley
½oz (15g) dried mixed berries
slice of lemon (optional)

Heat the olive oil in a small pan and sauté the shallot. Add the lentils, ginger, and garlic. Pour in the stock and simmer everything uncovered for around 15 minutes, until the lentils are just cooked.

Add the zucchini and bell pepper to the lentils and warm gently, adding a bit more water if necessary. Add the rosemary and season to taste with salt and pepper. Remove the lentils from the pan and leave to cool before pouring into a container. Pack the spinach leaves in a separate container.

To make the dressing, stir together the yogurt, harissa, and lemon juice, plus some salt and pepper. Pour the dressing into a jar and seal. Pack the topping ingredients in a separate container. Store the salad, dressing, and topping ingredients in the refrigerator until ready to serve.

AT WORK—Arrange the spinach on 2 plates and pour the lentils on top. If preferred, you can gently heat the lentil mixture beforehand. For the topping, pluck off the mint and parsley leaves, cut into strips, then add to the salad with the mixed berries, drizzling a dash of lemon juice over top, if desired. Add the dressing to the salad.

At home	At work	Serves	Kcal	Protein	Carbs	Fat
30 mins	5 mins	2	195	9g	23g	7g

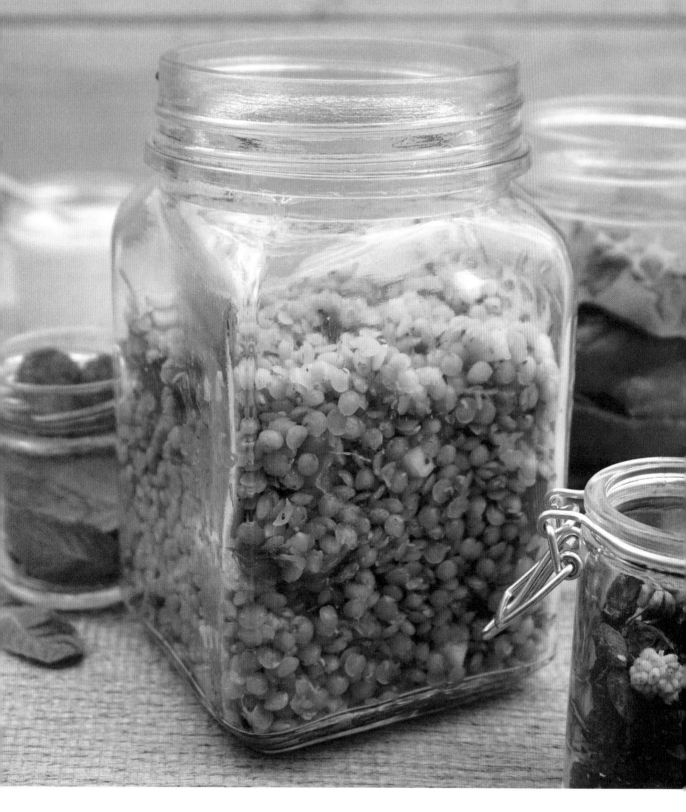

VEGETARIAN

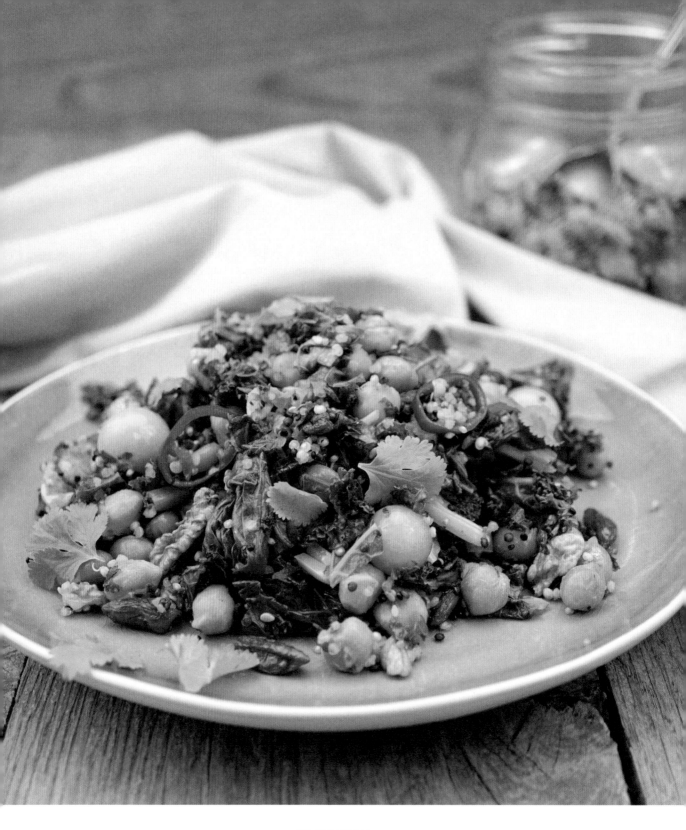

Kale and spinach salad

with an orange dressing

FOR THE SALAD

¾oz (20g) quinoa
1¾oz (50g) canned chickpeas
1 tbsp butter
1¾oz (50g) kale, stems removed
    and leaves chopped
1 garlic clove, finely chopped
¼ red chili, seeded and sliced
    into thin rings
¾oz (20g) walnuts, shelled and
    coarsely chopped
1 tsp goji berries, about 5g
6 cape gooseberries (physalis
    fruit), leaves removed
1¼oz (40g) spinach, stalks
    removed and leaves chopped
sprig of cilantro leaves

FOR THE DRESSING

2 tbsp orange juice
2 tbsp lemon juice
1 tsp agave syrup
salt

For the salad, wash the quinoa thoroughly in a strainer under running water. Cover with water in a small pan and simmer, uncovered, for 5–8 minutes, until just cooked. Rinse the chickpeas thoroughly in a strainer and leave to drain.

To make the dressing, stir together the orange juice, lemon juice, and agave syrup. Season the dressing to taste with salt. Drain the cooked quinoa in a strainer. Heat the butter in a large pan and sauté the kale until it wilts. Add the garlic and 1 tablespoon dressing and allow to cook briefly. Stir in the chickpeas and continue to cook everything for about another 5 minutes. Stir in the quinoa, chili, walnuts, goji berries, cape gooseberries, and spinach, and fry everything for 5 minutes. Add the cilantro leaves to the salad.

Transfer the salad from the pan into a jar and leave to cool. Pour any remaining dressing into a small jar. Close both jars and store in the refrigerator.

AT WORK—The salad can be eaten cold or warmed up slightly, as you prefer.

At home	At work	Serves	Kcal	Protein	Carbs	Fat
20 mins	5 mins	1	465	10g	28g	22g

Bell pepper boats
with cream cheese

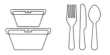

5½oz (150g) full-fat cream cheese
1 small tomato, seeds removed
    and flesh finely chopped
½ carrot, finely grated
½–¾in (1–2cm) piece of ginger,
    finely grated
juice of ½ lime
2–3 sprigs of chopped flat-leaf
    parsley leaves, plus extra
    to garnish (optional)
salt and freshly ground
    black pepper
6–8 colorful mini bell peppers,
    seeded and halved lengthwise

Combine the cream cheese in a bowl with the diced tomato, grated carrot, and ginger, add the lime juice, and mix everything thoroughly. Add the parsley to the cream cheese mixture, season with salt and pepper, and stir.

Pack the bell pepper halves and the cream cheese mixture in separate containers and seal. Store both in the refrigerator until ready to serve.

AT WORK—Arrange the bell pepper halves on two plates, skin-side down. Fill the bell pepper halves with the cream cheese mixture and, if desired, scatter some additional parsley over top.

At home	At work	Serves	Kcal	Protein	Carbs	Fat
15 mins	2 mins	2	230	7g	8g	19g

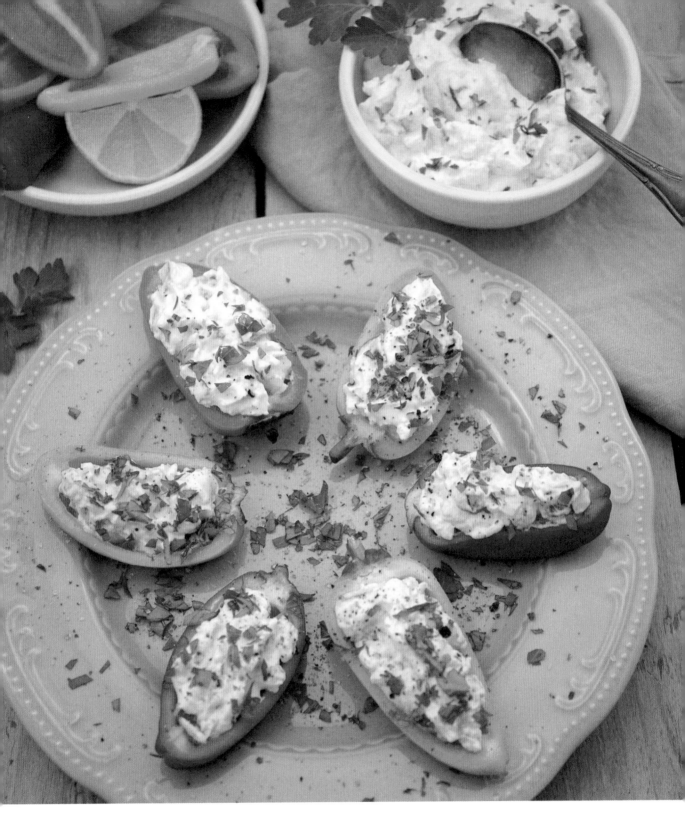

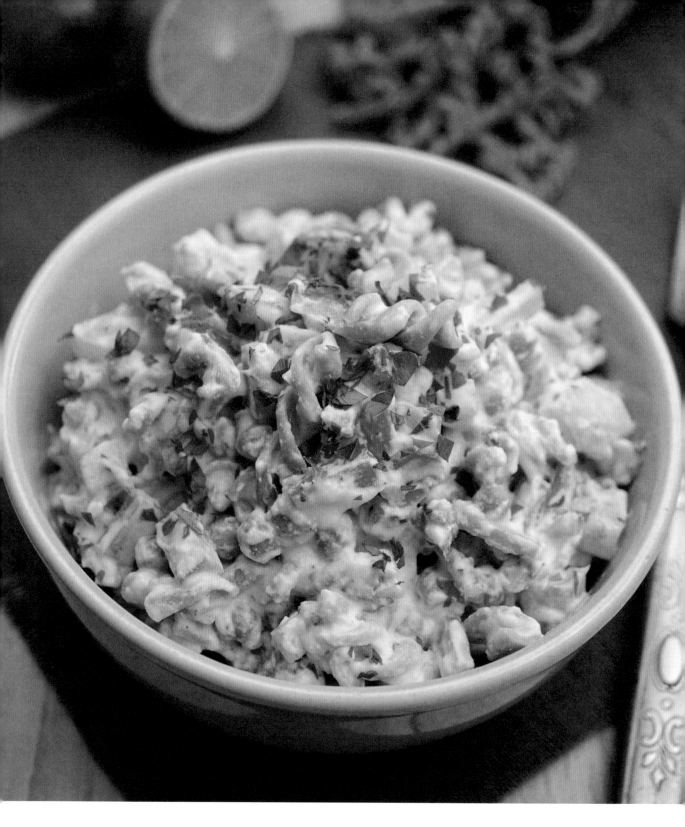

Chickpea pasta salad
with mixed vegetables

1¾oz (50g) chickpea pasta
  (such as chickpea fusilli from
  a health-food store)
salt and freshly ground
  black pepper
1¼oz (40g) carrots, cut into
  small pieces
1¾oz (50g) peas (freshly shelled
  or defrosted frozen ones)
1¾oz (50g) yellow bell pepper,
  seeded and cut into cubes
5¾oz (160g) yogurt
grated zest of 1 organic lime
3 sprigs of flat-leaf parsley
  leaves, chopped

Cook the chickpea pasta in a large pan of salted boiling water for 3 minutes, then add the carrots and peas and continue to simmer for about 3 minutes. Drain the pasta and vegetables in a strainer, rinse in cold water, and leave to drain.

In a bowl, mix the pasta and all the vegetables with the yogurt, lime zest, and parsley. Season the salad to taste with salt and pepper, transfer to a container, and seal. Store the salad in the refrigerator until ready to serve.

OUR TIP—The ingredients in this pasta salad can be varied and substituted to create endless different options. For example, it also tastes fantastic with dried tomatoes and arugula, or try adding some strips of roasted chicken breast and pieces of pineapple.

At home	At work	Serves	Kcal	Protein	Carbs	Fat
20 mins	0 min	1	225	16g	26g	6g

Zucchini pasta salad

with toasted pine nuts

1 tbsp walnuts, roughly
   chopped
1 tbsp pine nuts
1 small zucchini
1 tbsp lemon juice
1 tsp linseed
salt and freshly ground
   black pepper
1¾oz (50g) yellow bell pepper,
   seeded and cut into
   small cubes
1¾oz (50g) orange bell pepper,
   seeded and cut into
   small cubes
6 cherry tomatoes, halved

Toast the walnuts in a dry pan along with the pine nuts.

Use a spiralizer to turn the zucchini into long, thin noodles. Toss the zucchini noodles in a bowl with the lemon juice, walnuts, pine nuts, and linseed. Season the mixture with salt and pepper.

Transfer the zucchini noodles to a jar. Then layer up the bell pepper pieces and tomatoes on top. Close the jar and store the salad in the refrigerator until ready to serve.

OUR TIP—The zucchini salad can also be heated in a pan and eaten warm. To heat, simply add 1 tablespoon olive oil to the salad in the pan.

At home	At work	Serves	Kcal	Protein	Carbs	Fat
10 mins	0 min	1	180	7g	13g	11g

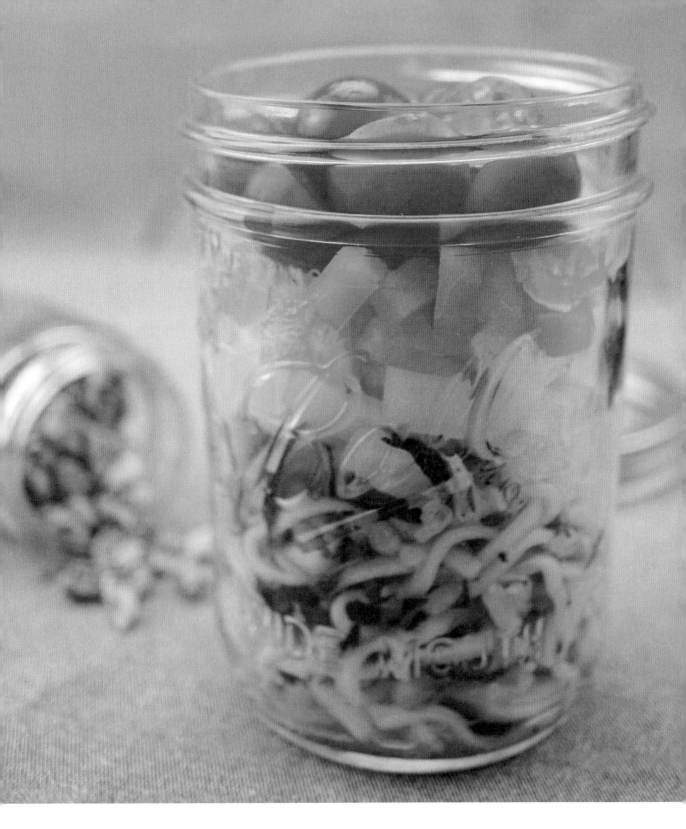

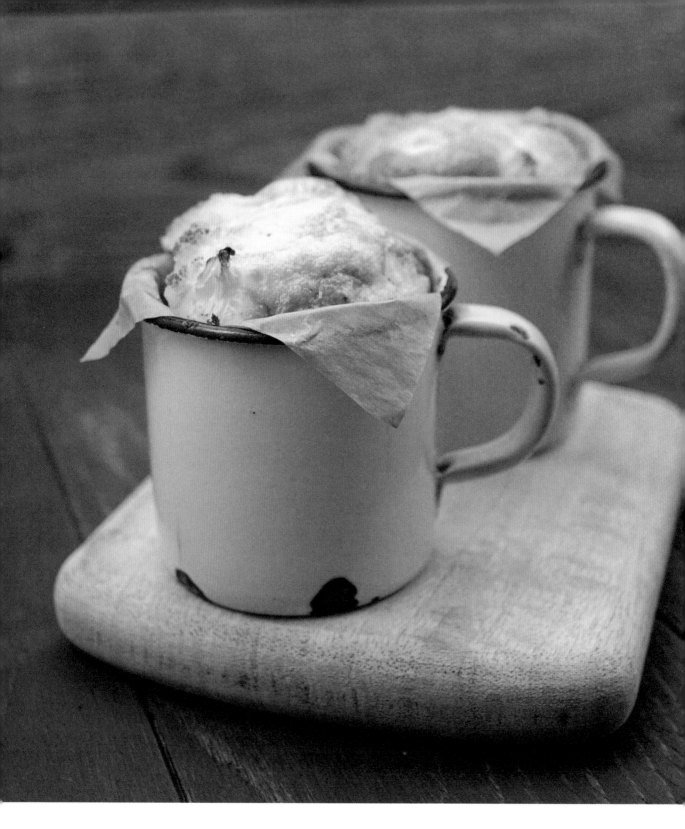

Cauliflower egg muffin
in a mug

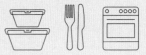

6 eggs
salt and freshly ground
   black pepper
7oz (200g) cauliflower florets

Preheat the oven to 475°F (240°C). Line 2 ovenproof mugs with parchment paper.

Whisk the eggs, then season with salt and pepper. Put the cauliflower florets into the mugs, pour the eggs over top, and bake in the center of the oven for 30 minutes.

Remove the mugs from the oven and leave the muffins to cool. Pack the muffins, still in their mugs, in a container and seal. Store the muffins in the refrigerator until ready to serve.

AT WORK—Preheat the oven to 425°F (220°C). Heat the cauliflower and egg muffins in their mugs in the oven for 15 minutes. The muffins can also be reheated in the microwave, just be sure your mugs are microwave safe. Heat the muffins all the way through.

OUR TIP—This recipe is also ideal as a quick "emergency fix"—just take eggs and your choice of vegetable to work and prepare on the spot. It tastes great with spinach, peppers, or mushrooms.

At home	At work	Serves	Kcal	Protein	Carbs	Fat
10 + 30 mins	15 mins	2	275	22g	5g	16g

Omelet rolls

with cream cheese filling

9½oz (280g) full-fat cream cheese
½ carrot, finely grated
1 tomato, finely diced
2 mini peppers, seeded,
   1 pepper cut into cubes, and
   1 pepper sliced into rings
½ red chili, seeded and finely
   chopped
juice of 1 lime
½–¾in (1–2cm) piece ginger,
   finely chopped
¼oz (10g) Parmesan cheese
salt and freshly ground
   black pepper
4 eggs
1 tsp olive oil

Mix the cream cheese with the carrot, tomato, diced pepper, chili, and lime juice. Add the ginger and grate in the Parmesan. Season the cream cheese mixture with salt and pepper and stir everything together once more.

Whisk the eggs in a bowl and season with salt and pepper. Heat half the olive oil in a pan and pour in half the egg mixture so that the base of the pan is covered. Let the omelet firm up briefly over medium heat, then flip it to finish cooking. Transfer the omelet from the pan onto a chopping board. Make a second omelet in the same way from the remaining egg mixture, and transfer this to the chopping board, too.

Spread the omelets with the cream cheese mixture, roll them up, transfer to a container, then seal. Pack the pepper rings in a separate container. Store the omelets and pepper rings in the refrigerator until ready to serve.

AT WORK——Place the omelets on a plate and serve with the pepper rings. If you wish, garnish with some lettuce, tomatoes, and herb leaves.

At home	At work	Serves	Kcal	Protein	Carbs	Fat
25 mins	1 min	2	595	26g	13g	49g

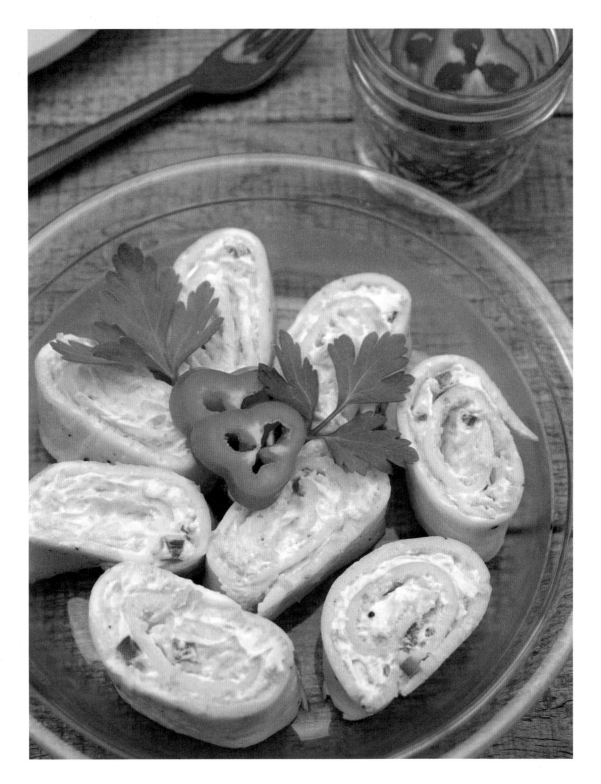

VEGETARIAN

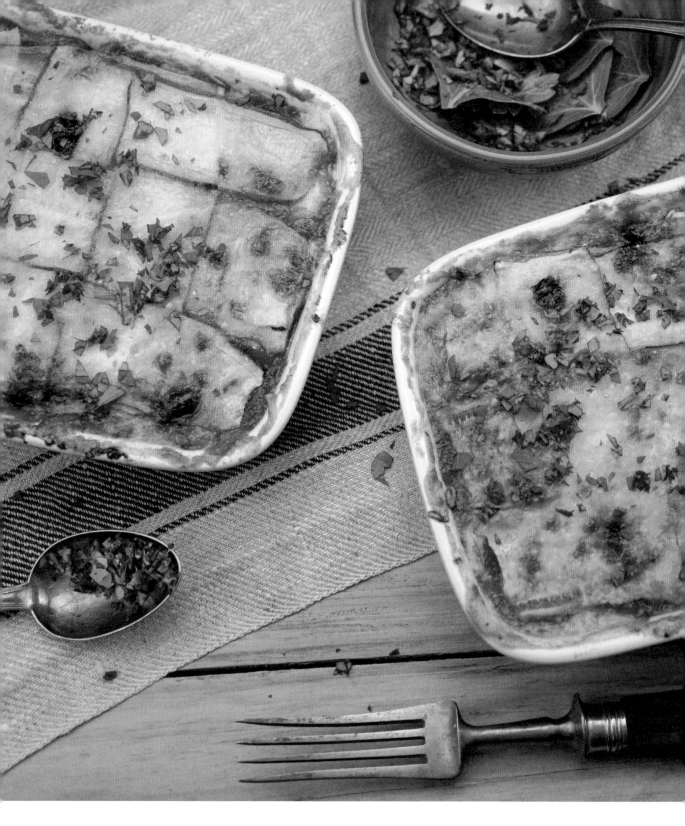

VEGETARIAN

Zucchini lasagna
the low-carb way

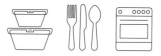

2 eggs
7oz (200g) ricotta
2oz (60g) grated Parmesan
   cheese, plus extra for sprinkling
grated zest of 1 organic lemon
salt and freshly ground
   black pepper
9oz (250g) canned chopped
   tomatoes
1 tsp dried thyme
1 tsp dried basil
1 zucchini, sliced lengthwise
   into strips with a peeler
7oz (200g) grated Gouda
chopped flat-leaf parsley,
   to garnish (optional)

Preheat the oven to 400°F (200°C). Whisk the eggs in a bowl. Stir in the ricotta, Parmesan, and lemon zest. Season the ricotta mixture with salt and pepper.

Stir the chopped tomatoes in a bowl with the thyme and basil, season the tomato sauce to taste with salt and pepper.

Arrange all the ingredients in alternating layers in 2 small ovenproof dishes (about 8 x 4in/20 x 10cm). Start with some zucchini strips, then some of the ricotta mixture, sprinkle on some of the Gouda, and spread some tomato sauce on top. Continue layering the ingredients in this manner, finishing with a layer of zucchini. Sprinkle on some Parmesan.

Bake the zucchini lasagnas in the center of the oven until golden brown. Remove from the oven and leave to cool in the dishes, then pack into containers. Store in the refrigerator until ready to eat. If you wish, pack some chopped parsley in a container.

AT WORK—Preheat the oven to 400°F (200°C) and reheat for about 15 minutes. Alternatively, reheat in the microwave until the lasagna is piping hot all the way through. Scatter with chopped parsley, if using.

At home	At work	Serves	Kcal	Protein	Carbs	Fat
30 + 30 mins	15 mins	2	780	58g	13g	48g

Stuffed mushrooms

with spinach and cream cheese

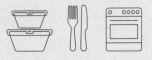

---

1 tbsp butter

1 shallot, finely diced

14oz (400g) mushrooms (preferably not too small), stalks removed and finely chopped, plus 2 whole mushrooms, finely chopped

1¼oz (40g) zucchini, cut into small cubes

1 garlic clove, crushed

1oz (30g) spinach leaves, finely chopped

2¼oz (70g) full-fat cream cheese

salt and freshly ground black pepper

¼oz (10g) Parmesan cheese, grated

Melt the butter in a pan and sauté the shallot. Add the chopped mushrooms and the zucchini. Add the garlic and the spinach and stir everything together. Add the cream cheese and let it melt. Season to taste with salt and pepper.

Preheat the oven to 425°F (220°C). Line a baking sheet with parchment paper. Place the mushroom caps upside down on the parchment paper and fill with the cream cheese mixture. Sprinkle on the Parmesan. Bake the mushrooms in the center of the oven for 15–20 minutes. Remove from the oven and leave to cool. Transfer to a container and close. Store the stuffed mushrooms in the refrigerator until ready to serve.

AT WORK—Preheat the oven to 425°F (220°C). Reheat the stuffed mushrooms in the oven for about 15 minutes. Alternatively, reheat in the microwave until the mushrooms are piping hot all the way through.

At home	At work	Serves	Kcal	Protein	Carbs	Fat
15 + 20 mins	15 mins	2	265	11g	4g	23g

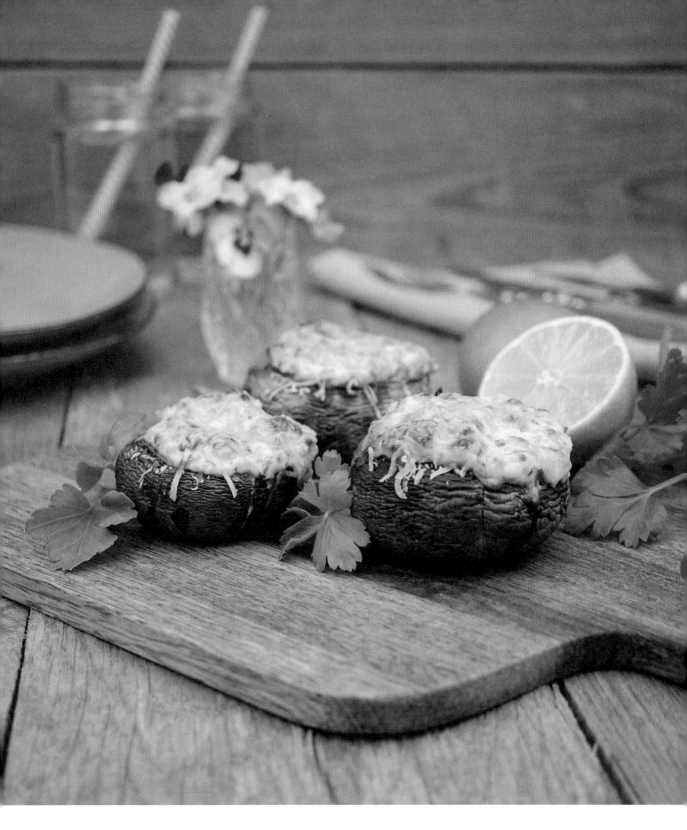

VEGETARIAN

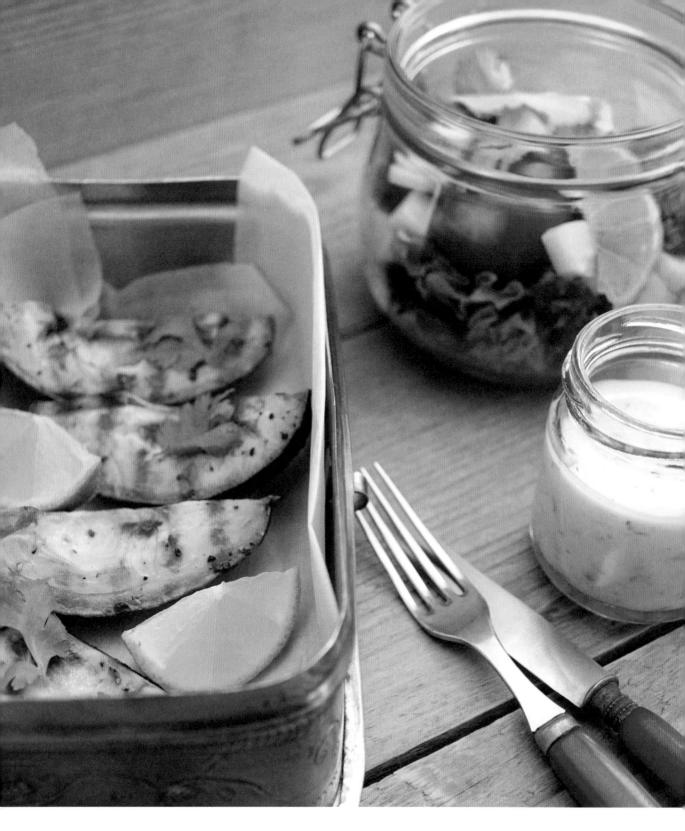

Grilled avocado with salad
and lime dressing

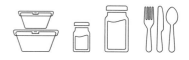

FOR THE SALAD
1oz (30g) mixed leaves
1 scant oz (25g) cucumber,
    peeled and chopped into
    small pieces
3 cherry tomatoes
slices of lime (optional)

FOR THE DRESSING
3oz (85g) yogurt
zest and juice of 1 organic lime
½ scallion, green section only,
    finely chopped
2 sprigs of cilantro leaves,
    finely chopped
salt and freshly ground
    black pepper
agave syrup (optional)

FOR THE AVOCADO
½ tbsp olive oil
1 avocado, pitted, flesh cut
    into 4 wedges
lime wedges (optional)

Place the salad ingredients in a jar, add some lime slices if you wish, and close the jar.

To make the dressing, put the yogurt in a bowl and stir in a dash of lime juice. Add the scallion, cilantro, and lime zest, and mix together thoroughly. Season the dressing with salt and pepper and some agave syrup, if using. Pour the dressing into a small jar and seal.

For the avocado, put the olive oil on a plate and season with salt and pepper, mixing them together with a fork. Toss the avocado slices in the oil mixture. Heat a griddle and fry the avocado slices, flesh side down, over high heat, until they have griddle marks. Transfer the avocado to a container, adding some extra lime wedges, if using. Store the dressing and the avocado in the refrigerator until ready to serve.

At home	At work	Serves	Kcal	Protein	Carbs	Fat
20 mins	0 min	1	310	6g	15g	24g

Pumpkin soup
with aromatic pumpkin seed oil

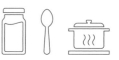

1¼oz (40g) butter
1 shallot, finely chopped
½ Hokkaido pumpkin (red kuri
   squash), peeled, seed removed,
   and cut into small pieces
7oz (200g) celeriac, cut into
   small pieces
½in (1cm) piece of ginger,
   peeled and finely chopped
3½fl oz (100ml) orange juice
1–2 tbsp lemon juice
salt and freshly ground
   black pepper
pumpkin seed oil, for drizzling

Melt the butter in a large pan and sauté the shallot briefly. Add the pumpkin and celeriac and sauté everything until golden. Deglaze the pan with a dash of water, then gradually add 1¼ pints (750ml) water. Add the ginger, cover, and simmer over moderate heat for 10–15 minutes, until the vegetables are soft.

Remove the pan from the heat and blend the soup using a hand-held blender. Add the orange and lemon juices and stir everything through once more. Season the soup to taste with salt and pepper, transfer it to a large jar, and leave it to cool. Close the jar and store the soup in the refrigerator until ready to serve.

AT WORK—Reheat the soup, but do not let it boil. Pour into bowls and drizzle with pumpkin seed oil.

OUR TIP—Chopped pumpkin seeds also make a great topping for this soup.

At home	At work	Serves	Kcal	Protein	Carbs	Fat
30 mins	10 mins	4	190	3g	18g	12g

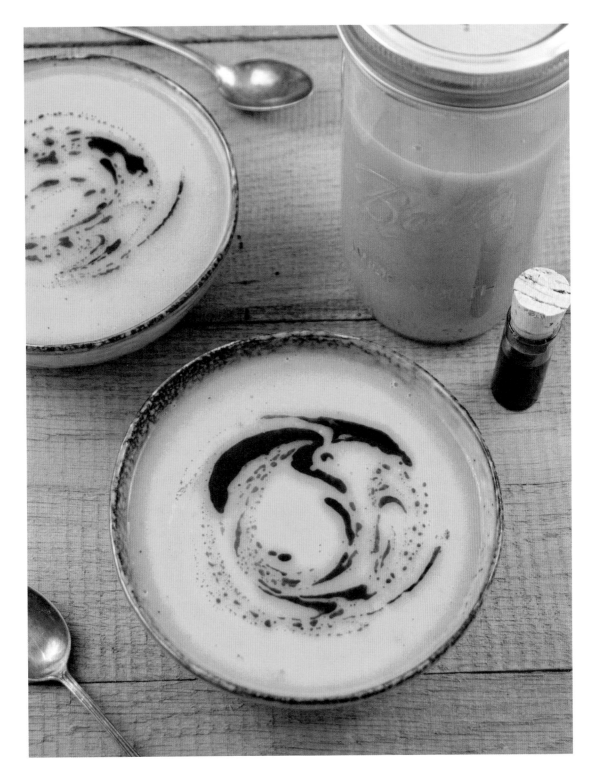

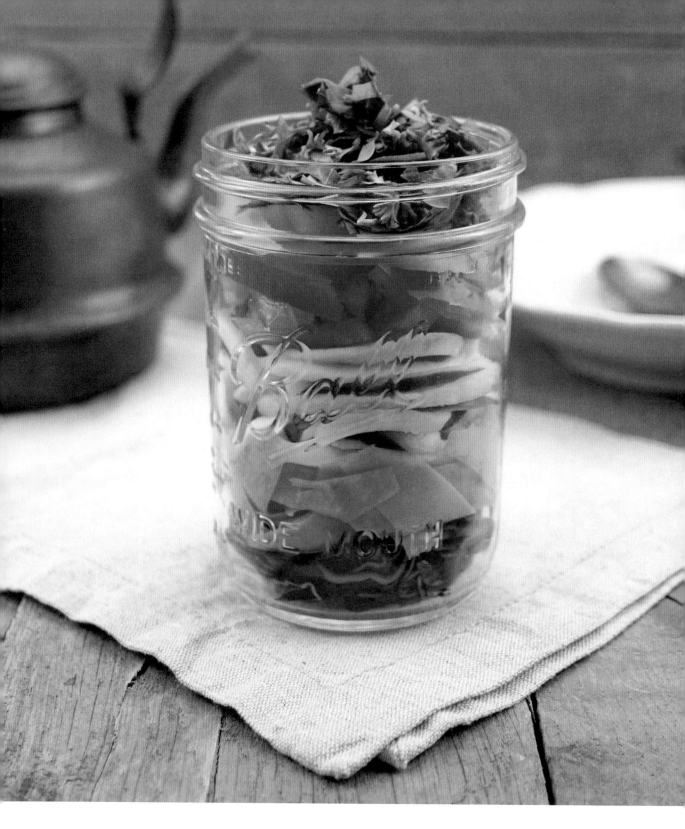

VEGETARIAN

Vegetable noodle soup

with fresh parsley

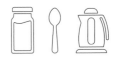

1¼oz (40g) zucchini
1 red cabbage leaf, about
    ½oz (15g)
¾oz (20g) squash or pumpkin
    flesh, thinly sliced
1¼oz (40g) red bell pepper,
    seeded and thinly sliced
1oz (30g) yellow bell pepper,
    seeded and thinly sliced
2 sprigs of flat-leaf parsley
    leaves, roughly chopped
salt and freshly ground black
    pepper (in lidded dispensers)

Using a spiralizer, slice the zucchini into long noodles. Wash the red cabbage and slice into thin strips.

Layer the red cabbage, pumpkin, zucchini, and both kinds of bell peppers in a jar. Finish with the parsley, then close the lid. Store the vegetable mixture in the refrigerator until ready to serve.

AT WORK—Fill the jar with boiling water and leave to steep for around 5 minutes with the lid on. Pour the soup into a deep dish and season with salt and pepper.

At home	At work	Serves	Kcal	Protein	Carbs	Fat
10 mins	6 mins	1	45	2g	8g	2g

Tomato and mozzarella kebabs

with herby yogurt

FOR THE KEBABS
5 cherry tomatoes, halved
1 mini cucumber, cut into discs
¼ yellow bell pepper, seeded
  and cut into ½in (1cm) cubes
sprig of basil leaves
5 mini mozzarella balls

FOR THE YOGURT
4–5 sprigs cilantro leaves,
  finely chopped
5½oz (150g) plain Greek
  yogurt (thick)
salt and freshly ground
  black pepper

ALSO
5 small wooden skewers

To make the kebabs, slide tomatoes, cucumber, bell pepper, basil leaves, and mozzarella balls onto the wooden skewers, alternating them. Put the kebabs into a container and seal.

For the yogurt, stir the cilantro into the yogurt. Season the herby mix to taste with salt and pepper. Pour into a container, then seal. Store the kebabs and herby yogurt in the refrigerator until ready to serve.

At home	At work	Serves	Kcal	Protein	Carbs	Fat
10 mins	0 min	1	238	19g	11g	13g

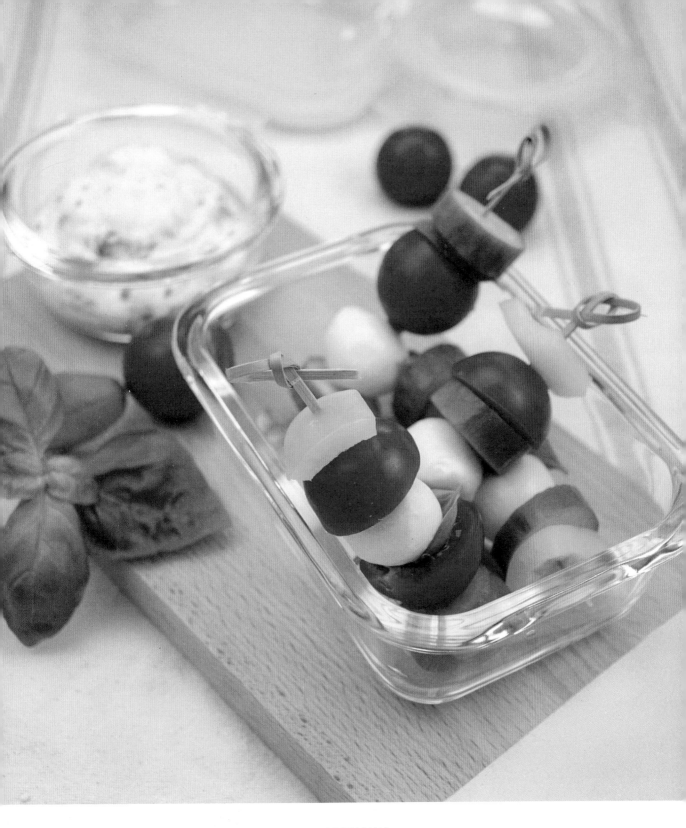

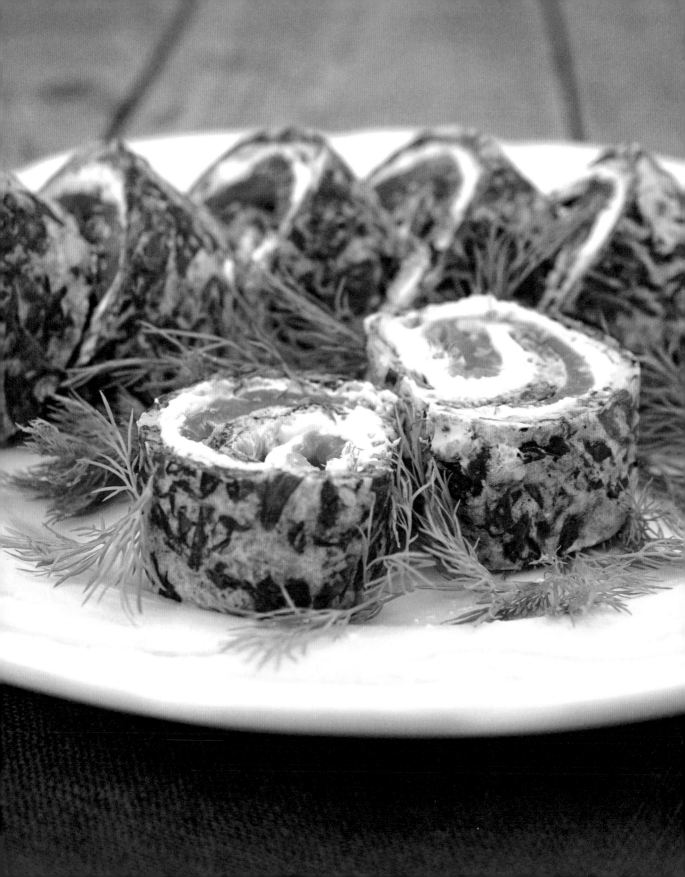

MEAT

AND FISH

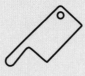

Chicken stock
with spices

1 chicken carcass
1 ¼in (3cm) piece of ginger, sliced
1 star anise
2–3 cinnamon sticks
salt

Place the chicken carcass in a saucepan with 7 pints (4l) water and bring to a boil. Add the ginger, star anise, cinnamon sticks, and salt, cover, and let everything simmer for 1 hour. Then add an additional 1¾ pints (1l) water and leave to simmer for 2 more hours.

Strain the chicken stock and pour immediately into sterilized, airtight bottles. Close the bottles immediately and stand them upside down for several minutes, then leave to cool. Alternatively, allow the stock to cool down, then freeze it in portions.

At home	At work	Serves	Kcal	Protein	Carbs	Fat
5 + 180 mins	0 min	4	—	—	—	—

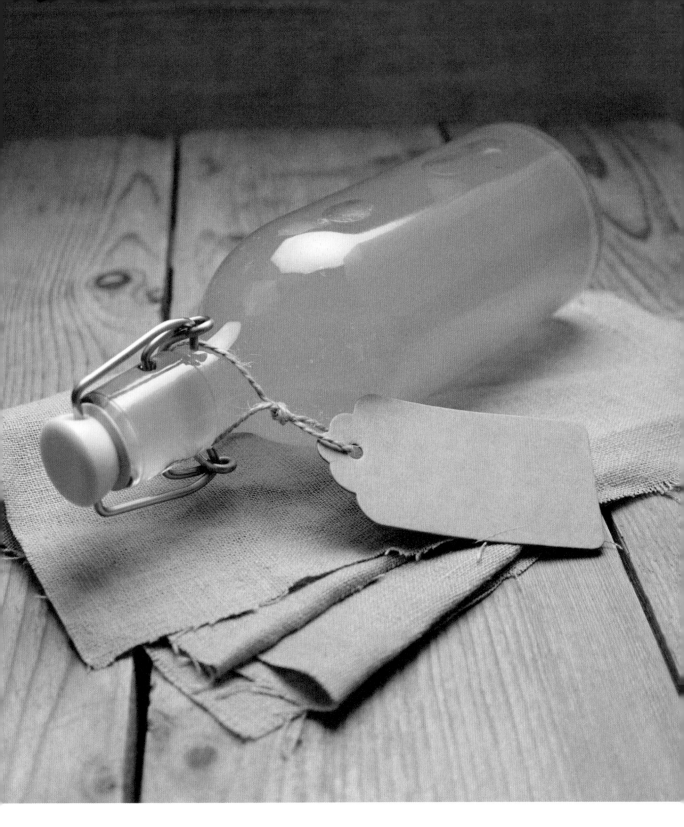

MEAT AND FISH

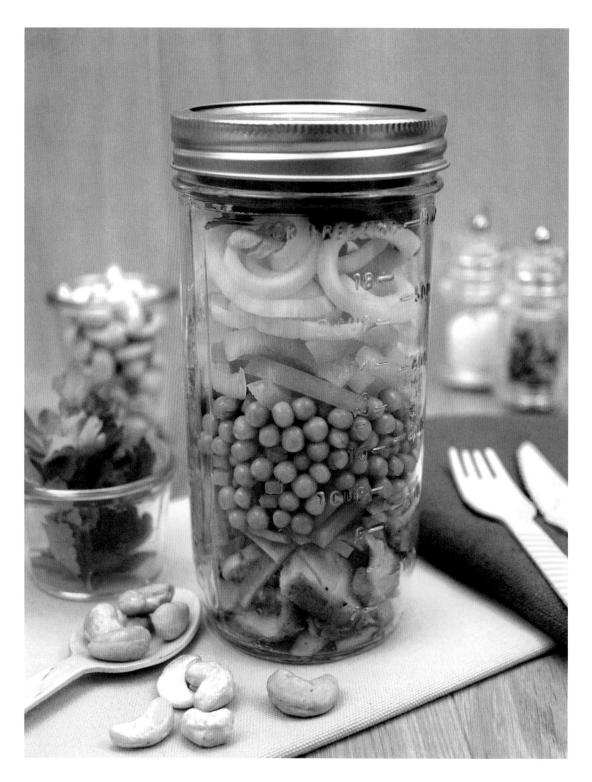

MEAT AND FISH

Life-enhancing soup
with chicken and cashew nuts

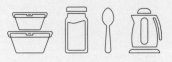

1 tbsp coconut oil
1 boneless chicken thigh
  (skin on), chopped into
  bite-sized pieces
1 broccoli stalk
1½oz (45g) carrot, cut into
  matchsticks
2oz (60g) peas (freshly shelled
  or defrosted frozen ones)
1¾oz (50g) yellow bell pepper,
  seeded and cut into
  matchsticks
2 sprigs of flat-leaf parsley
  leaves, chopped
1 tbsp cashews, roughly
  chopped
½ tsp ground cumin
½ star anise
salt and white pepper

Heat the coconut oil in a pan and sauté the chicken pieces for around 5–8 minutes, depending on their size, until cooked. Leave the meat to cool. Use a spiralizer to cut the broccoli stalk into thin noodles.

Layer the meat, carrot, peas, bell pepper, and broccoli one after the other in a jar and top with parsley and cashews. Seal the jar. Store the mixture in the refrigerator until ready to eat. Put the cumin and star anise plus some salt and pepper in a separate container.

AT WORK—Add the spice mixture to your jar and pour over boiling water. Close the jar and leave the soup to infuse for 5–7 minutes.

At home	At work	Serves	Kcal	Protein	Carbs	Fat
15 mins	7 mins	1	465	31g	18g	29g

Chicory salad
with chicken

1 tbsp olive oil
1¾oz (50g) chicken breast,
  cut into small pieces
salt and freshly ground
  black pepper
1 orange, divided into segments
1 chicory, thinly sliced
1–2 tbsp pomegranate seeds
handful of mixed leaves,
  roughly chopped
¼oz (10g) beet sprouts

Heat the olive oil in a pan and sauté the chicken pieces for 5–8 minutes, depending on their size, until cooked. Season with salt and pepper and leave to cool.

Layer the orange segments, chicory, pomegranate seeds, mixed leaves, chicken, and beet sprouts one after the other in a jar, then close it tightly. Store the salad in the refrigerator until ready to serve.

OUR TIP—Arrange the salad on a plate and drizzle with an aromatic oil, such as grapeseed or pumpkin seed oil.

At home	At work	Serves	Kcal	Protein	Carbs	Fat
15 mins	0 min	1	220	13g	12g	10g

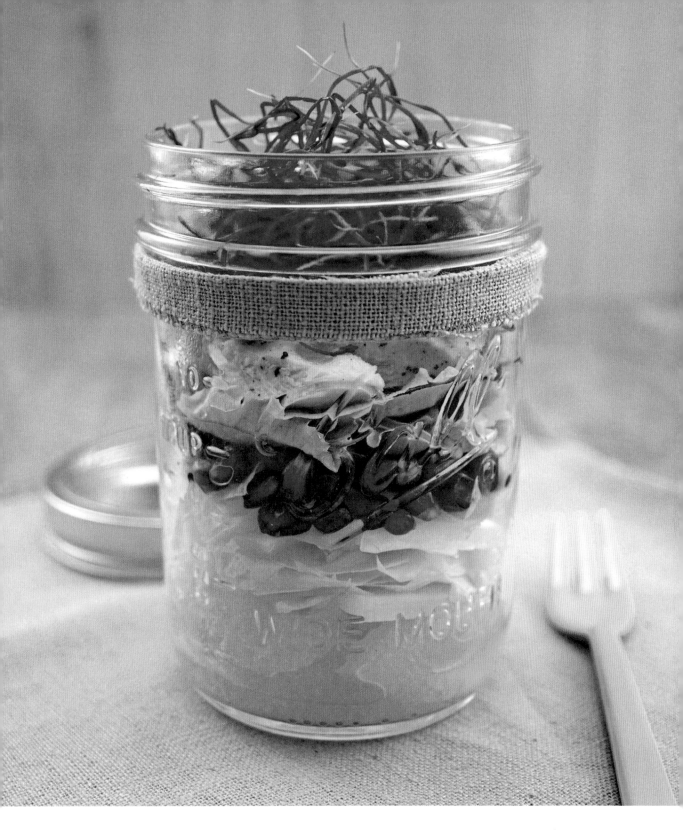

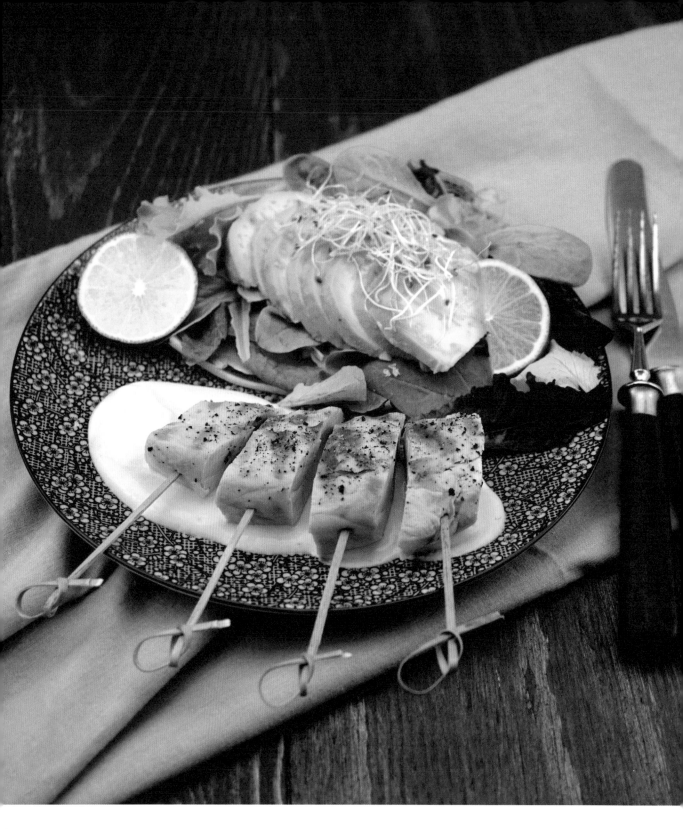

Chicken kebabs
with salad and mustard dressing

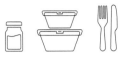

1 chicken breast, about
  5½oz (150g)
salt and freshly ground
  black pepper
½ avocado, pitted and
  flesh sliced
1–2 tsp lime juice
2 handfuls of mixed-leaf lettuce
1–2 tbsp alfalfa sprouts

FOR THE DRESSING
1 tbsp soy yogurt
½ tbsp plain Greek yogurt
  (thick)
1 tbsp lemon juice
½ tsp medium-hot mustard
salt

ALSO
4 small party skewers

Season the chicken breast with salt and pepper. Heat a pan and fry the chicken for around 5 minutes on each side, until it is cooked through and has acquired griddle marks. While the chicken is cooking, drizzle the avocado with lime juice.

To make the dressing, stir together both kinds of yogurt, lemon juice, and mustard. Season the dressing with salt, transfer it into a jar, and seal. Store the dressing in the refrigerator until ready to use.

Remove the chicken from the pan, slice into 4 pieces, leave to cool, then slide onto the party skewers. Put the skewers into a box and close. Put the lettuce, avocado, and sprouts into a separate box. Store everything in the refrigerator until ready to serve.

AT WORK—Arrange the lettuce on a plate with the avocado and alfalfa sprouts and season with salt and pepper. Put the dressing on the plate and arrange the chicken kebabs on top.

OUR TIP—If preferred, the chicken can be reheated briefly.

At home	At work	Serves	Kcal	Protein	Carbs	Fat
20 mins	5 mins	1	305	39g	6g	14g

Beef strips
Asian style

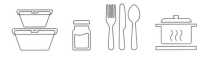

juice of ½ lime
1 tsp agave syrup
2 tbsp soy sauce
1 tbsp teriyaki sauce
1–2 tbsp sesame oil
5oz (140g) beef (suitable for frying, for example, fillet steak), sliced into bite-sized strips
1 carrot, cut into discs
1 bok choy, about 7oz (200g), quartered
2 mushrooms, thinly sliced
¼ cucumber, peeled, seeds removed, and thinly sliced
1oz (30g) rice noodles

FOR THE TOPPING
2 sprigs of cilantro leaves
1 tbsp chopped cashews
½ tsp white sesame seeds
½ tsp black sesame seeds

Stir together the lime juice, agave syrup, soy sauce, and teriyaki sauce in a little bowl. Heat the oil in a pan and sauté the beef, turning it regularly until brown all over. Add the carrot and bok choy and continue to fry briefly. Then add the mushrooms and cucumber and fry these briefly, too. Stir in the sauce mixture. Put the meat mixture into a container and seal. Leave to cool, then transfer to the refrigerator.

Add the cilantro leaves to a jar along with the cashews and sesame seeds. When taking this dish to work, bring the noodles with you in a container or in their packaging.

AT WORK—Prepare the rice noodles according to the instructions on the packaging. Heat the meat and vegetables in a pan, then stir in the hot noodles. Serve on a plate and scatter with cilantro, nuts, and sesame seeds.

OUR TIP—This recipe can also be prepared completely at home then served cold at work. Instead of rice noodles, you could also use low-carb noodles.

At home	At work	Serves	Kcal	Protein	Carbs	Fat
15 mins	10 mins	2	290	19g	24g	13g

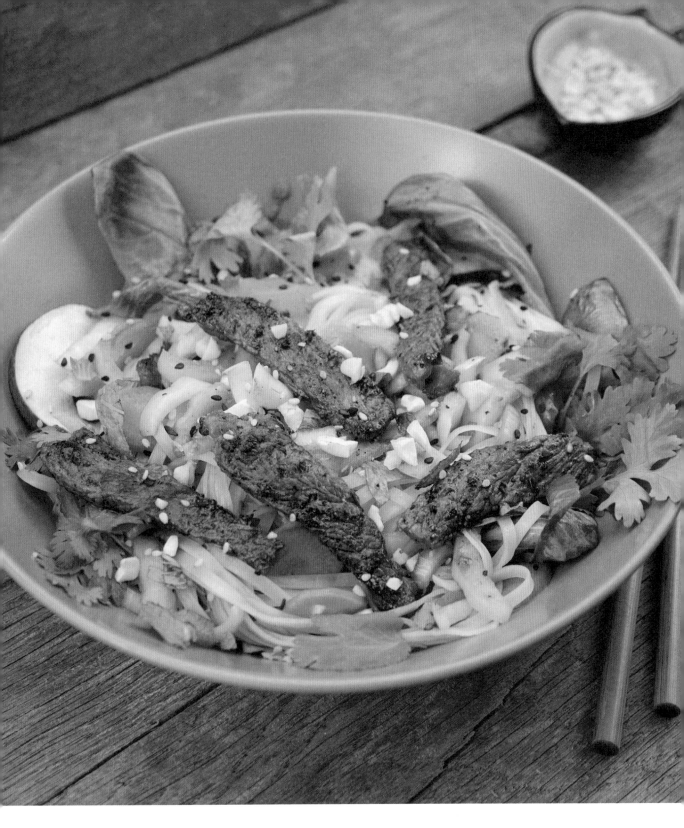

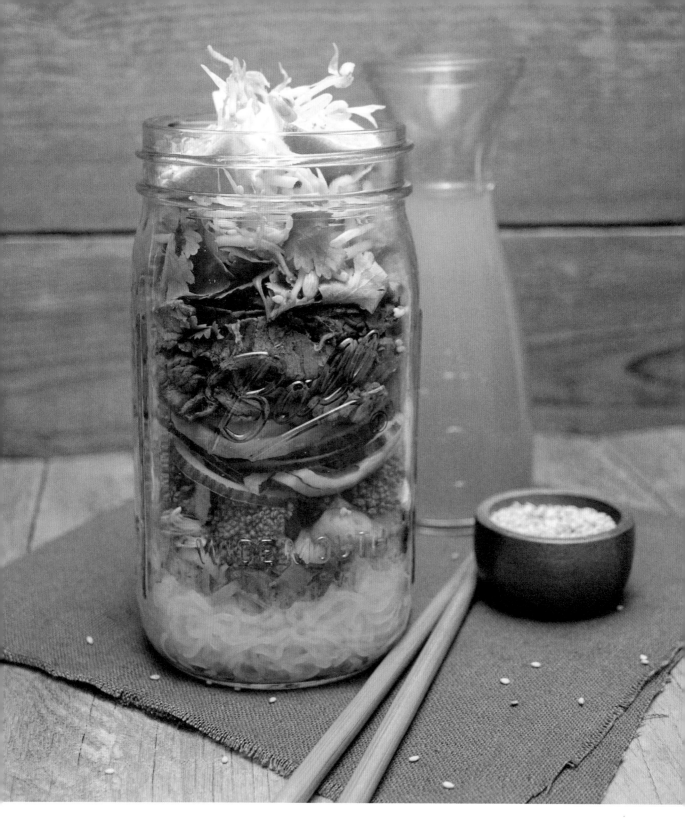

Asian noodle soup
with beef

3oz (85g) low-carb noodles
1 tbsp olive oil
2oz (60g) steak
salt and freshly ground
   black pepper
1 scallion, root discarded and
   white part thinly sliced
1 scant oz (25g) small broccoli
   florets
½ red onion, thinly sliced
1¾oz (50g) carrot, peeled
   into long "noodles"
2 sprigs of cilantro leaves
1–2 tbsp sprouts or shoots
   (whatever variety you like)
½ organic lime, sliced into
   wedges
16fl oz (500ml) chicken stock
   (see p. 129)
white sesame seeds for topping
   (optional)

Rinse off the noodles in a strainer with warm water and leave to drain. Heat the olive oil in a pan and sauté the beef until brown all over. Season the steak with salt and pepper, then slice into thin strips.

Layer the noodles, scallion, broccoli, red onion, carrots, steak, and cilantro in a tall jar, finishing with the sprouts or shoots and lime wedges. Close the jar and store the soup mixture in the refrigerator until ready to eat. Put the chicken stock and sesame seeds in separate jars. Store the chicken stock in the fridge.

AT WORK—Heat the chicken stock and pour it over the ingredients in the jar until everything is covered with stock. Close the jar and leave the soup to infuse for 5–8 minutes. Then pour the soup into a bowl and sprinkle with sesame seeds if desired.

At home	At work	Serves	Kcal	Protein	Carbs	Fat
15 mins	10 mins	1	230	16g	9g	7g

Rainbow rolls

with sweet and sour sauce

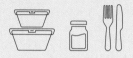

FOR THE SAUCE

pinch of agar agar powder

¼oz (5g) ginger, finely chopped

1 garlic clove, crushed

2 tsp sesame oil

3 tbsp cider vinegar

1 tsp lemon juice

1 tsp soy sauce

½ tsp tomato purée

1–2 tbsp agave syrup

½ tsp salt

FOR THE ROLLS

½ avocado, pitted, flesh sliced

1 organic lime

1¼oz (40g) cooked chicken

7oz (200g) low-carb noodles

¼ cucumber, cut into thin discs

¼ red bell pepper, seeded and
thinly sliced

¼ yellow bell pepper, seeded
and thinly sliced

1oz (30g) red cabbage leaves,
finely sliced

1 carrot, thinly sliced

1oz (30g) sugar snap peas

1 tbsp peas (freshly shelled or
defrosted frozen ones)

salt and white pepper

2 sprigs of mint leaves

2 sprigs of flat-leaf parsley leaves

9 sheets rice paper (6½in/16cm
diameter)

1 tbsp white sesame seeds

Stir the agar agar into 2 tablespoons cold water. Put the ginger, garlic, and agar agar water into a saucepan with the sesame oil, vinegar, lemon juice, and soy sauce, and bring to a boil. Add the tomato purée and 3–5 tablespoons of water and simmer for about 5 minutes. Season the sauce to taste with agave syrup and salt, transfer to a jar, and seal. Leave to cool. Drizzle the avocado with the juice of half the lime. Chop the cooked chicken into small pieces.

Prepare the noodles according to the instructions on the package and divide into 9 portions. Season the vegetables with salt and pepper. Mix the noodles with different combinations of vegetables, meat, and herbs. Fill a deep dish with water, soak each of the rice paper sheets for a couple of seconds, or as described in the instructions on the package, lay them on a plate, and let each become pliable. Roll up 1 of the noodle mixture portions in each sheet. Scatter the rolls with sesame seeds. Store in a container in the refrigerator, with some lime wedges cut from the remaining lime half, until ready to serve.

At home	At work	Serves	Kcal	Protein	Carbs	Fat
45 mins	0 min	9 pieces	80	2g	8g	4g

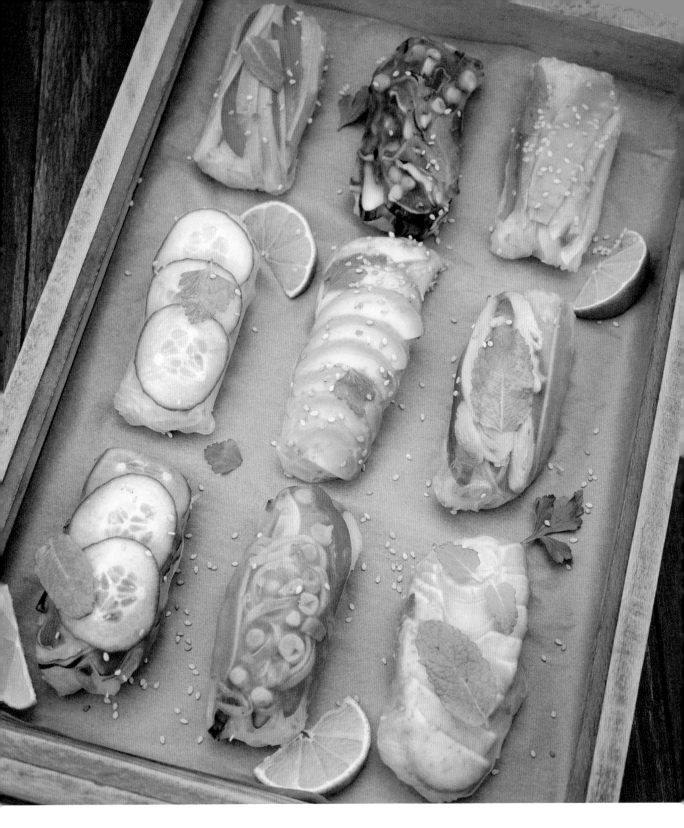

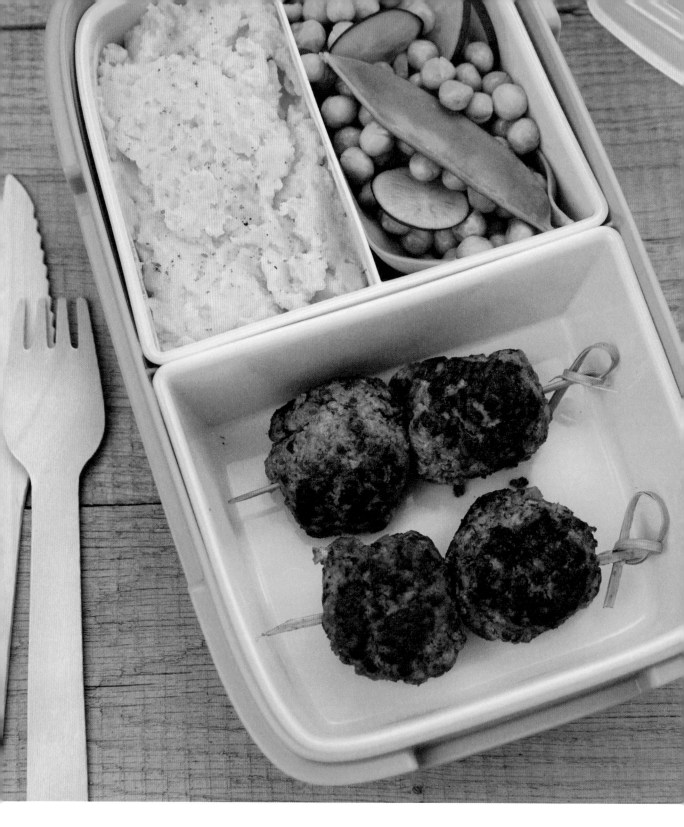

Meatballs with peas
and purée

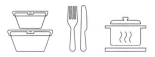

FOR THE MEATBALLS
1 tbsp butter
1 shallot, finely chopped
7oz (200g) ground beef
1 tsp capers, roughly chopped
1–2 sprigs of flat-leaf parsley
   leaves, roughly chopped
1 tbsp yogurt
1 tsp medium-hot mustard
1 egg yolk
salt and freshly ground
   black pepper
1 tbsp olive oil

FOR THE VEGETABLES
4 radishes, sliced
3oz (85g) sugar snap peas
3oz (85g) peas (freshly shelled
   or defrosted frozen ones)
½ tsp cider vinegar
dash of lemon juice

FOR THE PURÉE
1 small parsnip (about ¾oz/50g),
   chopped into small pieces
1 small sweet potato (about
   3½oz/100g), chopped into
   small pieces
freshly grated nutmeg

To make the meatballs, heat the butter in a pan and sauté the shallot until golden. Mix the ground beef in a bowl with the capers, shallot, parsley, yogurt, mustard, and egg yolk. Season the mixture with salt and pepper and shape into little balls. Heat the olive oil in the pan and fry the meatballs for 7–10 minutes, until brown, turning them occasionally. Leave the meatballs to cool and, if desired, slide them onto little party skewers.

Mix all the vegetables together in a bowl with the vinegar, lemon juice, and some salt and pepper.

For the purée, place the parsnip and sweet potato in a pan, barely cover with water, put the lid on, and cook for around 10 minutes, until soft. Drain the water. Use a masher to turn the vegetables into a purée, season with nutmeg and salt, and leave to cool. Pack up the meatballs, vegetables, and purée into separate containers and seal. Store everything in the refrigerator until ready to serve.

AT WORK—Reheat the meatballs and purée in the pan, then arrange on a plate. The vegetable mixture tastes great cold, or you can reheat it briefly, if preferred. The cold version is more crisp and contains more vital nutrients.

At home	At work	Serves	Kcal	Protein	Carbs	Fat
25 mins	10 mins	2	450	29g	21g	27g

Teriyaki chicken
with cauliflower rice

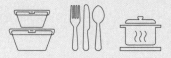

1 tsp coconut oil
1 chicken breast, about
    5¾oz (160g), cut into
    bite-sized pieces
1 garlic clove, crushed
3½ tbsp soy sauce
1 tsp honey
1 tbsp white sesame seeds
½ red onion, sliced into rings
½ red bell pepper, seeded and
    finely sliced
½ green bell pepper, seeded
    and finely sliced
3½oz (100g) Chinese cabbage,
    cut into ¾in (2cm) pieces
salt and freshly ground
    black pepper
½ cauliflower, about 14oz
    (400g), finely grated to
    make "rice"
1 tsp black sesame seeds
2 sprigs of cilantro

Heat the coconut oil in a pan and toss in the chicken strips. Sauté on all sides until they are cooked through and have browned slightly. Add the garlic to the pan, along with the soy sauce, honey, and white sesame seeds, and sauté briefly. Add the onion, bell peppers, and Chinese cabbage and continue to fry everything for 5–10 more minutes, stirring occasionally. Season the teriyaki chicken with salt and pepper, transfer to a container, and leave to cool. Seal the container.

Mix the grated cauliflower rice with the black sesame seeds, transfer to a container, and seal. Pack the cilantro in a separate container. Keep all the containers in the refrigerator.

AT WORK—Put the cauliflower rice into a bowl. Heat the teriyaki chicken with the vegetables and arrange on 2 plates. Wash the cilantro and shake it dry, pluck off the leaves, and sprinkle over the teriyaki chicken.

At home	At work	Serves	Kcal	Protein	Carbs	Fat
15 mins	10 mins	2	295	28g	13g	13g

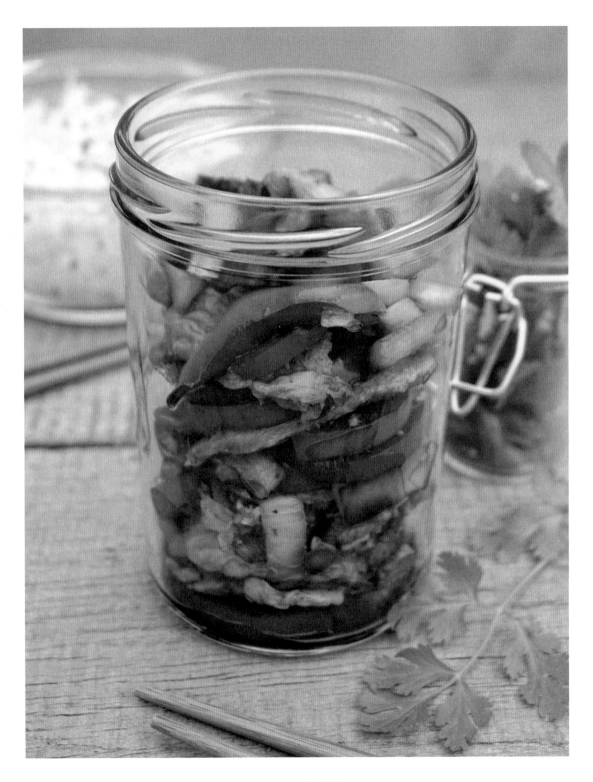

MEAT AND FISH

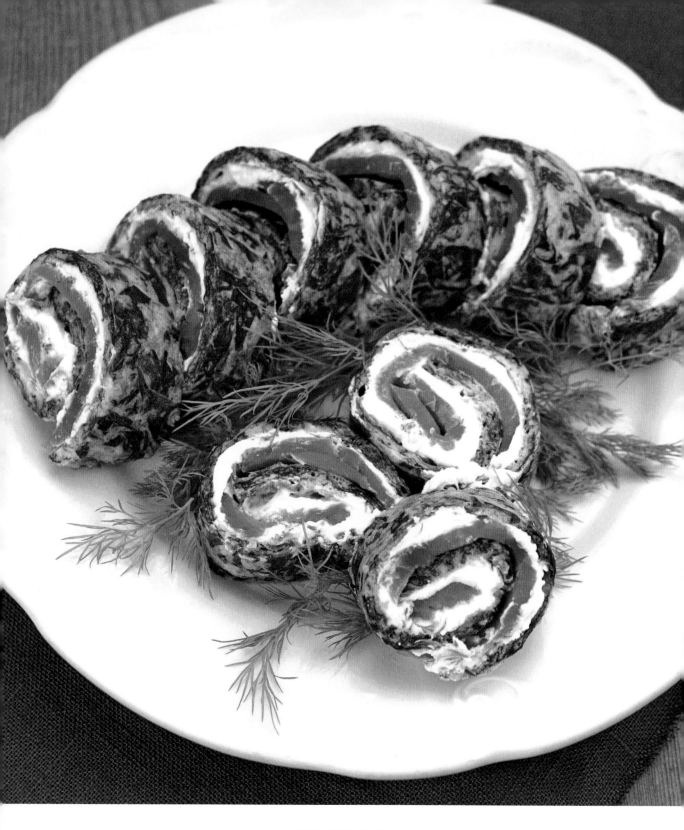

Spinach wraps
with smoked salmon and horseradish

FOR THE WRAPS
9oz (250g) spinach
3 eggs
pinch of grated nutmeg
salt and freshly ground
    black pepper
1½oz (45g) grated Parmesan
    cheese

FOR THE FILLING
½oz (150g) full-fat cream cheese
zest and juice of 1 organic lemon
½in (1cm) piece of ginger,
    finely grated
1 tsp horseradish
salt
3–4 sprigs of dill leaves
5½oz (150g) wild smoked
    salmon

Put the spinach into a steamer over a small amount of water and steam for 3–5 minutes. Remove the steamer from the pan containing the water, quickly run some cold water through the spinach, and leave to drain.

Preheat the oven to 350°F (180°C). Line a baking sheet with parchment paper. Using a hand-held whisk, beat the eggs with the nutmeg and some salt and pepper in a bowl until they are foamy. Stir in the Parmesan and then the spinach. Spread the egg mixture over the parchment paper to create a rectangle and bake in the center of the oven for 15–20 minutes. Remove the wrap from the oven and leave to cool.

While the egg is cooking, stir together the cream cheese, lemon zest, ginger, horseradish, some lemon juice, and salt.

Spread the wrap with the cream cheese mixture, sprinkle on the dill, and place the salmon on top. Roll everything up carefully and wrap the roll in plastic wrap to help it keep its shape. Pack into a container and store in the refrigerator.

AT WORK—Slice the wrap using a sharp knife, wiping the knife with a clean, dry cloth after each cut.

At home	At work	Serves	Kcal	Protein	Carbs	Fat
30 mins	1 min	4	295	21g	3g	22g

Pan-fried shrimp

with cucumber and pineapple salad and mango chutney

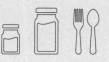

FOR THE CHUTNEY

2 tbsp low-calorie sweetener
  such as stevia
½in (1cm) piece of ginger,
  finely chopped
½ red chili, seeded and finely
  chopped
juice of 1 lime
1 tbsp cider vinegar
½ mango, finely chopped

FOR THE SALAD

2 cucumbers, about 2lb 5oz
  (600g), seeded and finely
  chopped
1 medium pineapple, about
  2lb 5oz (600g), cored and
  finely chopped
4 sprigs of cilantro leaves,
  roughly chopped
4 tbsp lime juice
salt and freshly ground
  black pepper
16 shrimp (heads removed,
  shells on)
4 tbsp olive oil

Heat the sweetener in a pan until it becomes liquid. Add the ginger and chili, deglaze with the lime and vinegar mixture, then simmer everything for a few minutes. Add the mango pieces and leave the chutney to simmer for around 30 minutes, stirring regularly. If it becomes too dry, add some water. Transfer the chutney to a jar and seal. Leave to cool.

For the salad, combine the cucumbers, pineapple, cilantro, and lime juice in a bowl. Season with salt and decant into jars.

Peel the shrimp, make an incision along the backs, and remove the intestine. Wash and dab the shrimp to dry. Heat the oil in a pan, fry the shrimp briefly on all sides, and season with salt and pepper. Leave the shrimp to cool, then add them to the salad and seal the jars. Store the salads in the refrigerator until ready to serve.

At home	At work	Serves	Kcal	Protein	Carbs	Fat
60 mins	0 min	4	247	15g	18g	10g

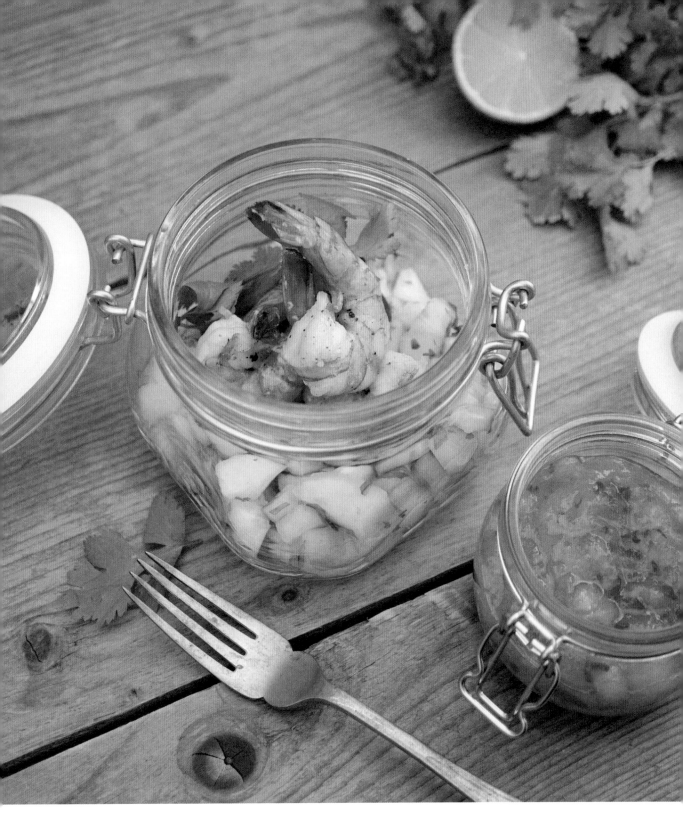

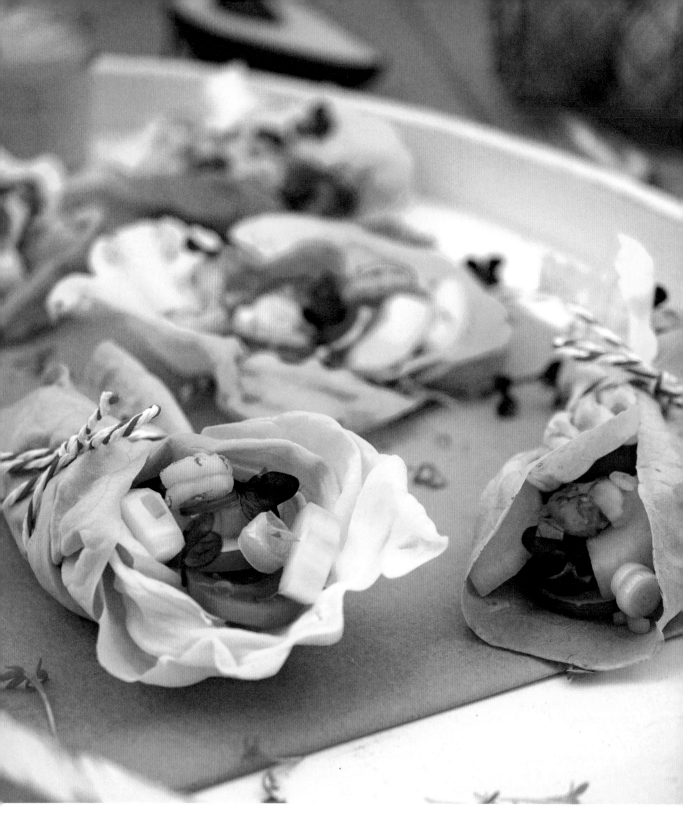

Salad wraps with shrimp
and avocado cream

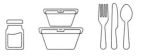

FOR THE SALAD
5 cherry tomatoes
3 radishes
¼ cucumber, peeled
    and chopped into
    bite-sized pieces
½ scallion, root discarded, white
    part sliced into thin rings
1 chili, seeded and finely sliced
4½oz (125g) shrimp, cooked
    and peeled
1 tbsp cress (such as garden
    cress or red radish cress), cut
zest and juice of 1 organic lemon
8 large round lettuce leaves

FOR THE CREAM
½ avocado, pitted
juice of ½ lime
2 sprigs of cilantro leaves
3 sprigs of dill leaves
3 tbsp yogurt
salt and freshly ground
    black pepper

Put the first seven salad ingredients into a bowl. Add the zest and 1 tablespoon lemon juice and mix everything together. Transfer the mix to a container. Pack the lettuce leaves in a separate container. Seal the containers and store them in the refrigerator.

To make the cream, add the avocado flesh to a blender beaker along with the lime juice. Add the herbs and yogurt to the avocado and process with a hand-held blender until it becomes a smooth purée. Season the creamy mix with salt and pepper to taste, transfer to a jar, and seal. Store the cream in the refrigerator until ready to use.

AT WORK—Lay the lettuce leaves out on a plate and distribute the shrimp salad between them, seasoning to taste with salt and pepper. Add the avocado cream to the wraps. If desired, tie up the wraps with some baker's twine.

At home	At work	Serves	Kcal	Protein	Carbs	Fat
10 mins	2 mins	3	95	8g	4g	5g

Fish cakes

with pear, fennel, and pea salad

FOR THE SALAD

½ fennel bulb, about 4½oz
  (125g), finely sliced
½ small pear, about 2oz (60g),
  peeled, cored, and thinly
  sliced
¼ scallion, thinly sliced
3½oz (100g) peas (freshly
  shelled or defrosted
  frozen ones)
2 sprigs of dill leaves, chopped
2 sprigs of cilantro leaves,
  chopped
grated zest of ½ organic lemon
1 tbsp lemon juice
2 tbsp orange juice
salt and freshly ground
  black pepper

FOR THE FISH CAKES

8oz (225g) salmon fillet, skin
  removed, cut into small cubes
1 shallot, finely diced
½in (1cm) piece of ginger,
  grated
½ chili, seeded and finely
  chopped
3 sprigs of dill tips, chopped
grated zest of ½ organic lemon
1 tbsp lime juice (or lemon juice)
1 egg yolk
1 tbsp olive oil

To make the salad, combine the fennel, pear, scallion, peas, herbs, and lemon zest in a salad bowl. Stir in the lemon and orange juices. Season the salad to taste with salt and pepper, transfer to a jar, and seal. Store the salad in the refrigerator until ready to eat.

To make the fish cakes, combine the salmon, shallot, ginger, chili, dill, lemon zest, lime juice, and egg yolk in a bowl, and season the mixture with salt and pepper. Heat the oil in a pan. Shape 4 fish cakes, all the same size, from the salmon mixture and fry them in the pan for about 8 minutes, until brown all over, turning them once during cooking. Let them cool, pack them in a container, and store in the refrigerator until ready to serve.

AT WORK—Reheat the fish cakes in a pan and arrange them on a plate with the salad.

At home	At work	Serves	Kcal	Protein	Carbs	Fat
20 mins	10 mins	2	395	30g	15g	18g

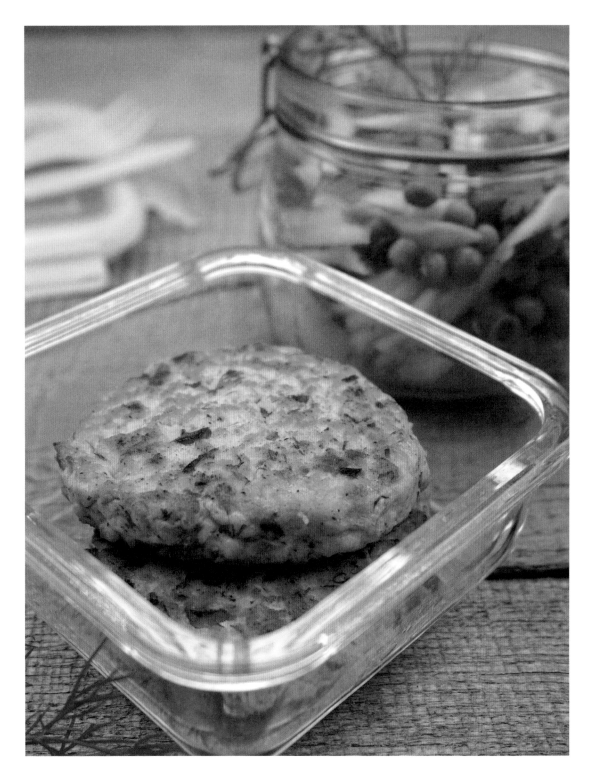

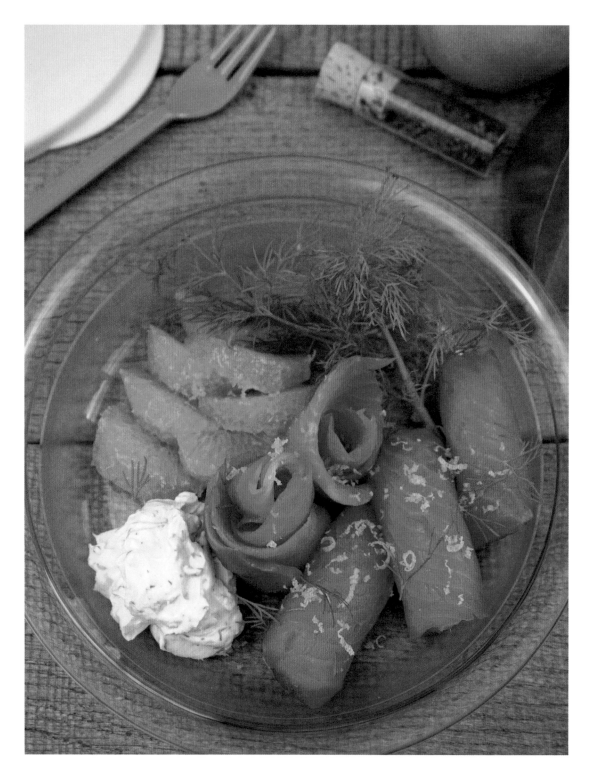

MEAT AND FISH

Fish platter

with gravlax

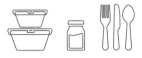

FOR THE DIP

2 sprigs of dill tips, finely
    chopped
1¾oz (50g) goat's milk
    cream cheese
½ tsp wasabi paste
zest and juice of 1 organic
    lemon

FOR THE GRAVLAX

3½oz (100g) salmon
2–3 sprigs of dill tips
1 mandarin orange, pith
    removed and fruit cut into
    segments
salt and freshly ground black
    pepper (in lidded dispensers)
chili flakes
zest of 1 organic lemon

To make the dip, combine the dill, cream cheese, and wasabi.
Stir the lemon zest and some of the juice into the cheese
mixture. Season the dip with salt and pepper, transfer to
a jar, and seal. Store in the refrigerator until ready to use.

For the gravlax, pack up all the ingredients in containers, then
store the salmon in the refrigerator until ready to serve.

AT WORK—To prepare the gravlax, arrange the salmon on
a plate with the dill and the mandarin. Sprinkle the salmon with
salt, pepper, chili flakes, and lemon zest, and add the dip.

At home	At work	Serves	Kcal	Protein	Carbs	Fat
10 mins	5 mins	1	365	26g	9g	24g

Tuna and egg salad
with homemade mayo

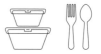

FOR THE SALAD

4 eggs

4½oz (130g) can of tuna
  in brine (drained weight)

1¾oz (50g) cornichons or dill
  gherkins, finely chopped, plus
  3 tbsp pickling liquid

½ scallion, finely sliced

1 celery stalk, finely sliced

2oz (60g) fennel, finely
  chopped

2 radishes, finely chopped

1oz (30g) yellow bell pepper,
  seeded and finely chopped

1oz (30g) red bell pepper,
  seeded and finely chopped

1 tbsp cider vinegar

3½oz (100g) yogurt

salt and freshly ground
  black pepper

FOR THE MAYONNAISE

1 egg yolk

1 tsp medium-hot mustard

1 tsp lemon juice

4fl oz (120ml) oil

FOR THE TOPPING

4 radishes, thinly sliced

2 sprigs of curly-leaf parsley,
  leaves roughly chopped

4 tsp radish cress

To make the salad, hard boil the eggs in boiling water for 10 minutes, run under cold water, peel, and chop into little pieces. Let the tuna drain in a strainer, then mash it with a fork.

For the mayonnaise, stir together the egg yolk, mustard, and lemon juice in a bowl with a whisk. Gradually add the oil, one drop at a time at first, then in a thin stream, mixing everything thoroughly until you have a creamy mayonnaise. Season with salt and pepper.

Stir together the tuna, eggs, vegetables, vinegar, and 3 tablespoons of the pickling liquid in a bowl. Mix in the yogurt and mayonnaise. Season the salad to taste with salt and pepper, transfer to a container, and seal.

Put the ingredients for the topping into a container. Store the salad and topping in the refrigerator until ready to serve.

AT WORK— If you wish, portion the salad into little bowls. Add the topping ingredients to the salad.

At home	At work	Serves	Kcal	Protein	Carbs	Fat
20 mins	0 min	4	430	14g	4g	39g

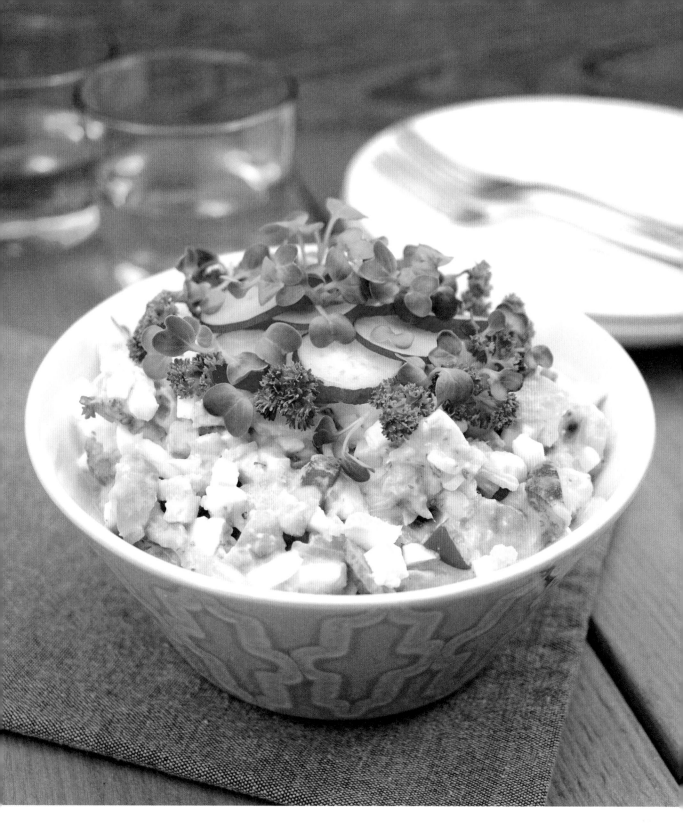

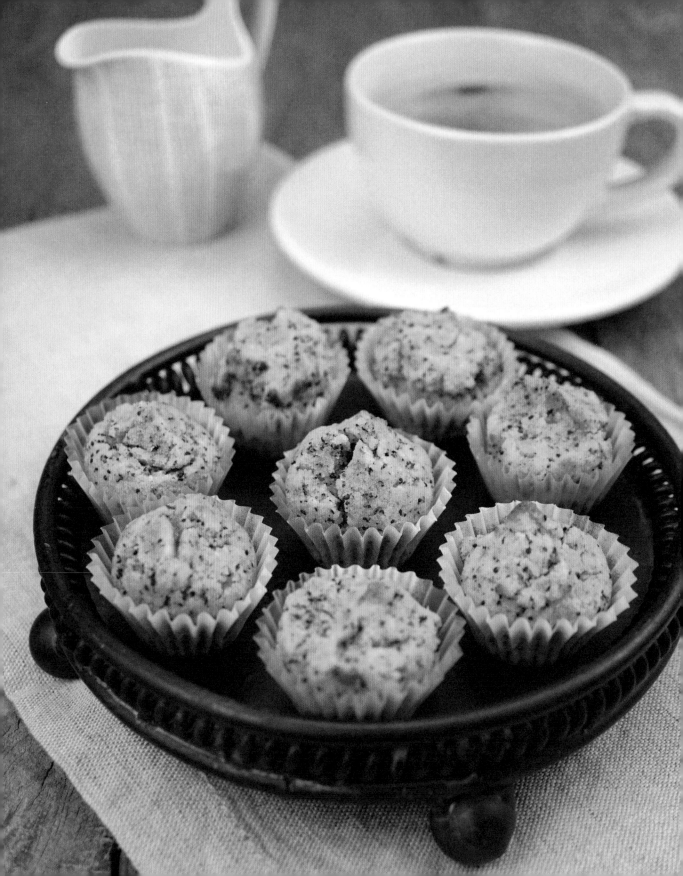

SNACKS

AND CAKES

Low-carb energy bars
with nuts

1oz (30g) walnuts
2oz (60g) almonds
1½oz (45g) pumpkin seeds
3 dates, pitted
1 tbsp cranberries
1 scant oz (25g) sunflower seeds
seeds from 1 vanilla bean
½ tsp salt
1 heaped tbsp coconut flour

Preheat the oven to 300°F (150°C). Line a baking sheet with parchment paper. Roughly chop the walnuts, almonds, and pumpkin seeds in a food processor, then add the dates and cranberries and chop those, too. Combine the nut mixture with the sunflower seeds, vanilla, salt, and coconut flour, kneading for several minutes until you obtain a malleable consistency. Shape the mixture into 6 bars, approximately ½in (1cm) thick, and place on the sheet. Bake in the center of the oven for 20–30 minutes, until golden brown. Let cool, then store in a tin.

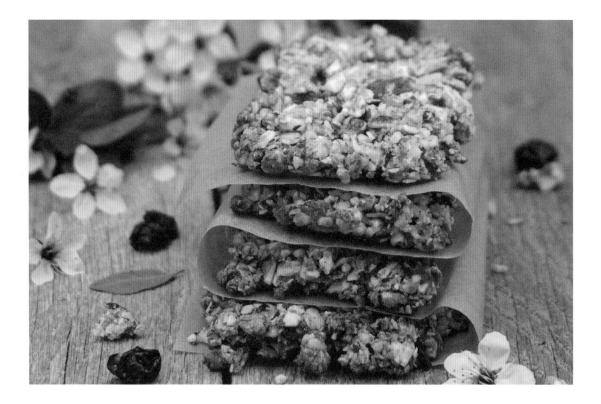

At home	At work	Serves	Kcal	Protein	Carbs	Fat
15 + 30 mins	0 min	6	185	7g	7g	13g

Sesame bars

power snack

½oz (15g) fine oat flakes
2½oz 75g) dates, pitted
¼oz (10g) ground almonds
¼oz (10g) sliced almonds
¾oz 20g) white sesame seeds
1oz (30g) cashew butter
(see p. 56)

Lightly toast the oats in a dry pan. Blend the dates in a food processor to create a purée. Use your hands to knead the oats, processed dates, almonds, sesame seeds, and cashew butter to create a dough. Place the dough on a sheet of parchment paper, cover with a second sheet of parchment paper, and roll out to a thickness of approximately ¼in (5mm) using a rolling pin. Cut into 6 bars and let them firm up in the refrigerator. The bars will keep refrigerated in a container for at least 10 days.

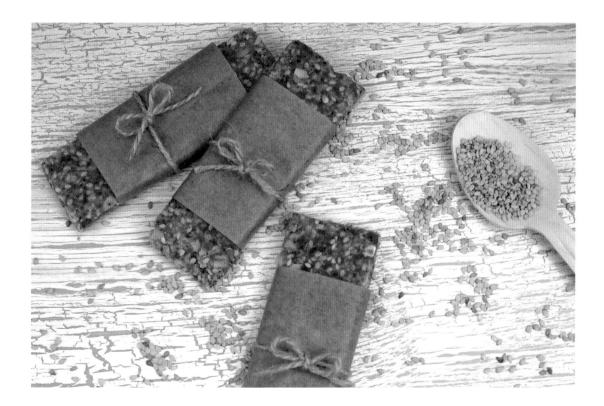

At home	At work	Serves	Kcal	Protein	Carbs	Fat
10 mins	0 min	6	120	3g	12g	6g

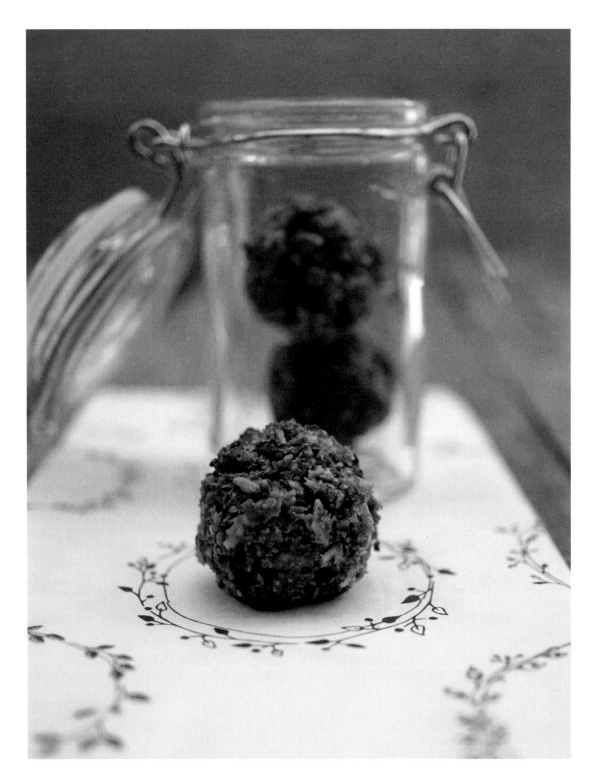

Energy balls

with coconut and vanilla

1oz (30g) spelt bran
¾oz (20g) ground almonds
½oz (15g) sliced almonds
¼oz (10g) chia seeds
½ tsp vanilla powder
1 tbsp cocoa nibs
½oz (15g) coconut sugar
¼oz (10g) coconut flakes
¾oz (20g) smooth coconut oil
2½ tbsp double cream or
   heavy cream
1 tbsp maple syrup

Preheat the oven to 375°F (190°C). Line a baking sheet with parchment paper. Place the spelt bran and ground almonds in a bowl. Crumble the sliced almonds by hand into the spelt mixture and add the chia seeds, vanilla, cocoa nibs, coconut sugar, and coconut flakes. Mix everything together.

In a separate bowl, combine the coconut oil, cream, and maple syrup. Add this mixture to the dry spelt mixture and stir everything well.

Shape the mixture into walnut-sized balls with your hands and place them on the parchment paper. Bake the balls in the center of the oven for around 10 minutes, until golden brown.

Remove from the oven and allow the balls to cool down on the sheet. Store in the refrigerator in a sealed tin or jar. Refrigerated, the balls will keep for around 2 weeks.

At home	At work	Serves	Kcal	Protein	Carbs	Fat
15 + 10 mins	0 min	12	75	2g	3g	6g

Fruit slices
in four flavors

BASIC RECIPE
2 tbsp ground nuts
2 tbsp dried fruit
6 round wafer papers or edible
    rice paper (2in/5cm diameter)

BERRY SLICES
2 tbsp ground hazelnuts
1 tbsp fine oat flakes
2 tbsp dried berries
1 date, pitted

APRICOT SLICES
2 tbsp ground almonds
3 dried apricots
1 date, pitted

APPLE CINNAMON SLICES
2 tbsp ground almonds
1 tbsp flaked almonds
1 tbsp coconut chips
4 dried apple rings
½ tsp ground cinnamon

PLUM AND COCOA SLICES
2 tbsp ground almonds
3 prunes
1 tsp raw cocoa powder
1 tsp cocoa nibs
1 date, pitted

Put all the dry ingredients for one recipe into a food processor and chop finely. Add 2 tablespoons of water and mix everything thoroughly again. Place the wafer paper discs next to each other on your work surface.

Use your hand to shape 3 balls from the fruit mixture. Press each of the balls onto a wafer paper and place a second wafer paper disc on top. Press the balls flat so that they are all the same size and the fruit mixture creates an even layer over the entire disc. The fruit slices will keep for several days in an airtight container.

OUR TIP—The fruit slices will taste even better if prepared with fruit juice instead of water. If you have a sweet tooth, you could sweeten them to taste with agave syrup or any other kind of natural sweetener.

OUR IDEAS FOR OTHER DELICIOUS FLAVORS—Mango and ginger, fig and sesame, date and peanut, or cranberry and coconut.

At home	At work	Serves	Kcal	Protein	Carbs	Fat
10 mins	0 min	3	105	3g	8g	6g

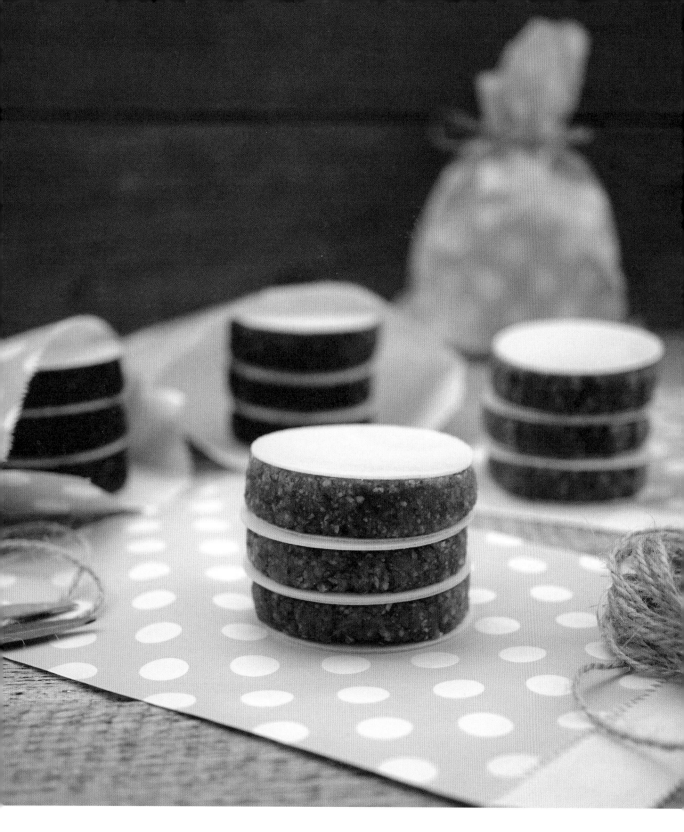

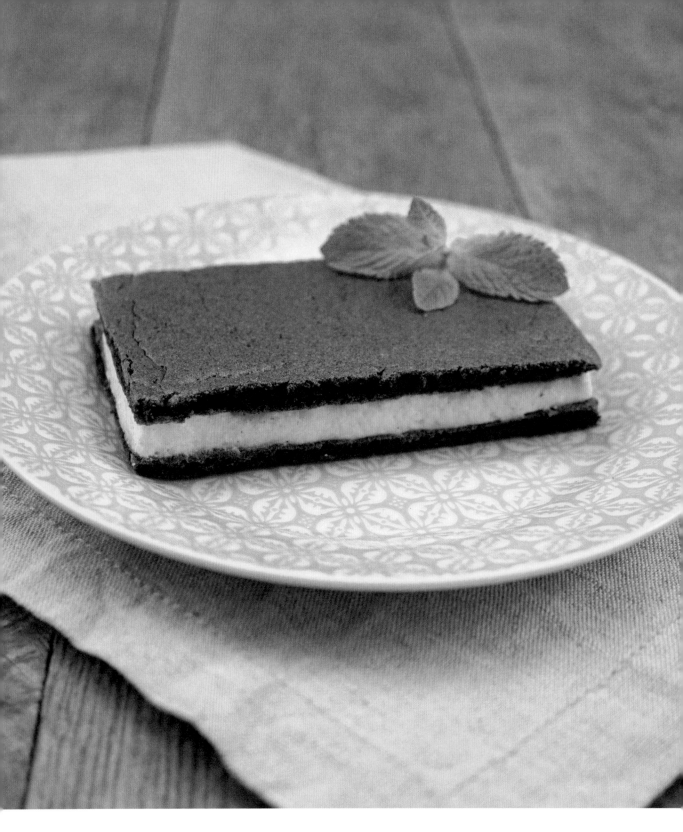

Cream-filled sandwich cookie
the low-carb way

FOR THE CHOCOLATE COOKIE
1 egg
5g raw cocoa powder
1 scant oz (25g) full-fat
 cream cheese

FOR THE FILLING
1 very fresh egg white
1 scant oz (25g) plain Greek
 yogurt (thick)
1 scant oz (25g) mascarpone
1 tbsp coconut protein powder
pinch of vanilla powder

Preheat the oven to 400°F (200°C). Line a baking sheet with parchment paper. To make the dough, separate the egg yolk from the white. Use a hand-held whisk to beat the egg white in a bowl until stiff. In a separate bowl, stir together the egg yolk, cocoa, and cream cheese. Carefully fold the beaten egg white into this mixture.

Spread the mixture out evenly on the parchment paper to create a rectangle measuring about 4 x 8in (10 x 20cm), and bake in the center of the oven for around 10 minutes. Remove from the oven and leave to cool.

To make the cream filling, beat the egg white until stiff. Combine the yogurt and mascarpone in a bowl. Stir in the protein powder and vanilla. Fold the beaten egg white into the cream and leave the mixture to stand briefly.

Cut 2 equal-sized rectangles from the chocolate slab. Put the cream on one rectangle and spread it out evenly. Place the second rectangle on top of the cream and press down slightly. Put the sandwich cookie into a tin and seal. Store in the refrigerator until ready to eat.

OUR TIP —If the low-carb sandwich cookie is being prepared in the evening and won't be eaten until the following day, we recommend waiting to spread on the cream until just before you are ready to eat.

At home	At work	Serves	Kcal	Protein	Carbs	Fat
20 + 10 mins	0 min	1	371	35g	5g	24g

Apple and orange muffins
with quinoa

1¾oz (50g) quinoa
3½oz (100g) coconut oil
1¾oz (50g) low-calorie
   sweetener such as stevia
1 egg
3½oz (100g) spelt flour with
   a high gluten content
2½oz (75g) whole meal
   spelt flour
1 scant oz (25g) coconut flour
1 tsp cream of tartar
5–7fl oz (150–200ml) almond
   milk (see p.22, or store-bought)
2 small apples, peeled,
   cored, and chopped into
   small pieces
1 orange, pith removed and fruit
   chopped into small pieces

ALSO
1 x 12-cup muffin pan
12 paper muffin liners

Preheat the oven to 400°F (200°C). Rinse the quinoa in a strainer under running water. Transfer it to a small pan, cover with water, and simmer uncovered for 8–10 minutes, until soft. Insert a paper liner into each of the cups in the muffin pan.

Melt the coconut oil in a pan over a low heat. Place the sweetener, egg, and quinoa in a bowl and stir in the melted coconut oil. In a separate bowl, combine both types of spelt flour, the coconut flour, and cream of tartar. Add the flour mixture to the coconut oil and egg mixture. Using a hand-held whisk, gradually beat in enough almond milk to create a thick batter. Finally, fold in the apple and orange pieces with a spoon. Distribute the batter evenly between the paper liners.

Bake the muffins in the center of the oven for 20 minutes. Then insert a wooden skewer to see if they are done; as long as no batter sticks to the inserted skewer, the muffins are ready. Otherwise, cook for around 5 minutes longer. Remove from the oven and leave the muffins to cool for about 5 minutes in the pan. Then lift them out and allow to cool on a wire rack. Pack them up in a container to take with you.

At home	At work	Serves	Kcal	Protein	Carbs	Fat
20 + 25 mins	0 min	12	167	4g	13g	10g

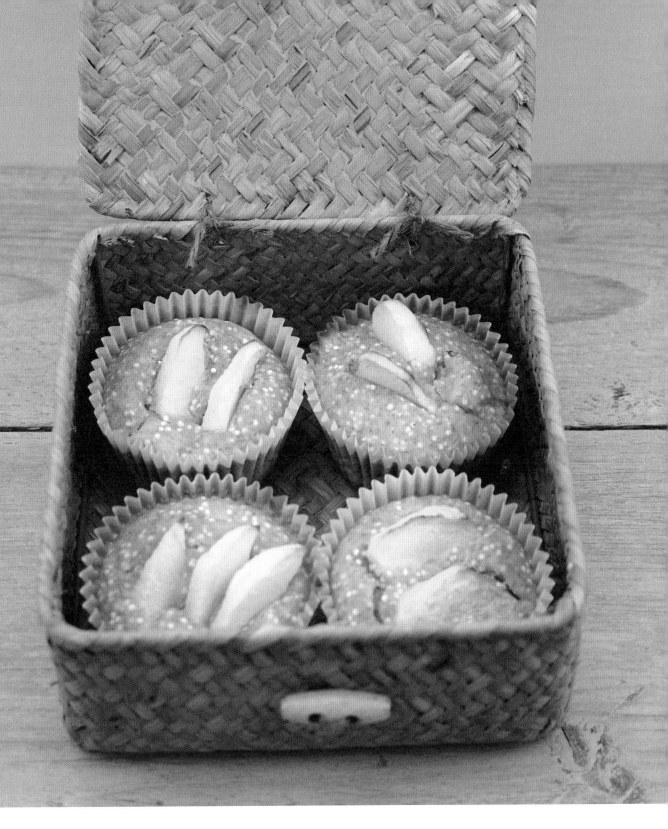

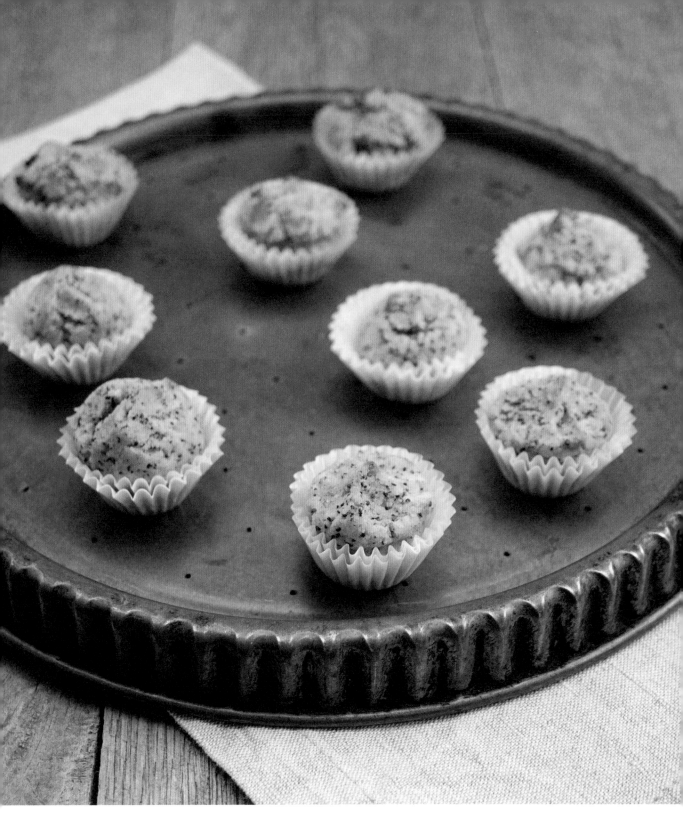

Mini muffins
with poppy seeds and lemon

1½oz (45g) butter
grated zest of 2 organic lemons
2 eggs
1oz (30g) coconut flour
½oz (15g) low-calorie
    sweetener such as stevia
1 tbsp poppy seeds
pinch of baking soda
pinch of vanilla powder
pinch of ground turmeric
pinch of salt

ALSO
32 mini muffin paper cases

Preheat the oven to 375°F (190°C). Double up the muffin liners one inside another so that you end up with 16 sets. Put them on a baking sheet. Melt the butter in a small pan over low heat, then stir in the lemon zest.

Place the eggs, coconut flour, sweetener, poppy seeds, baking soda, vanilla, turmeric, and salt in a bowl, and stir in the butter mixture with a wooden spoon.

Pour an even quantity of the mixture in the paper liners, using around 1 tbsp for each muffin. Bake the muffins in the center of the oven for 5 minutes. Then lower the oven temperature to 275–300°F (160–170°C) and bake the muffins for an additional 5–8 minutes, until done.

Remove the muffins from the baking sheet and leave to cool on a wire rack. Pack them up in a container to take with you.

OUR TIP—The lemon flavor in the muffins will be particularly enhanced if the citrus is zested immediately before adding the zest to the warm butter.

At home	At work	Serves	Kcal	Protein	Carbs	Fat
10 + 13 mins	0 min	16	45	2g	1g	4g

Blueberry vanilla cake

for a sweet morning treat

1¾oz (50g) butter
2–3 tbsp blueberries (fresh
　or frozen)
2 eggs
¾oz (20g) low-calorie
　sweetener such xylitol
1oz (30g) light low-calorie
　sweetener such as erythritol
3oz (85g) almond flour
½ tsp cream of tartar
1 tsp vanilla powder
2oz (60g) coconut fat (the
　firm layer from a can of
　coconut milk)
low-carb substitute for
　confectioner's sugar
　(optional)
edible flowers (optional)

ALSO
1 springform pan
　(6½–7in/16–18cm diameter)
shortening to grease the pan

Preheat the oven to 400°F (200°C). Grease the springform pan. Melt the butter in a small pan over low heat. Wash the fresh blueberries and leave to drain.

Using a hand-held whisk, beat the eggs in a bowl until they are foamy. Add the sweeteners and whisk everything until pale and creamy.

Combine the almond flour, cream of tartar, and vanilla in a large bowl. Add the butter and coconut fat and stir. Fold in the egg and sweetener mixture. Finally, add the blueberries to the mix (there is no need to defrost frozen berries) and stir everything through once more.

Transfer the mixture to the springform pan and bake in the center of the oven for 30 minutes. Test with a wooden skewer to see if it is done; as long as none of the mixture sticks to the inserted skewer, the cake is ready. Otherwise, continue to cook for 10–15 minutes longer.

Remove from the oven and allow the cake to rest in the pan for around 10 minutes. Release the cake from the pan and leave to cool on a wire rack. Dust with the confectioner's sugar substitute, if using, and decorate with edible flowers, if using.

At home	At work	Serves	Kcal	Protein	Carbs	Fat
15 + 45 mins	0 min	8	130	6g	3g	9g

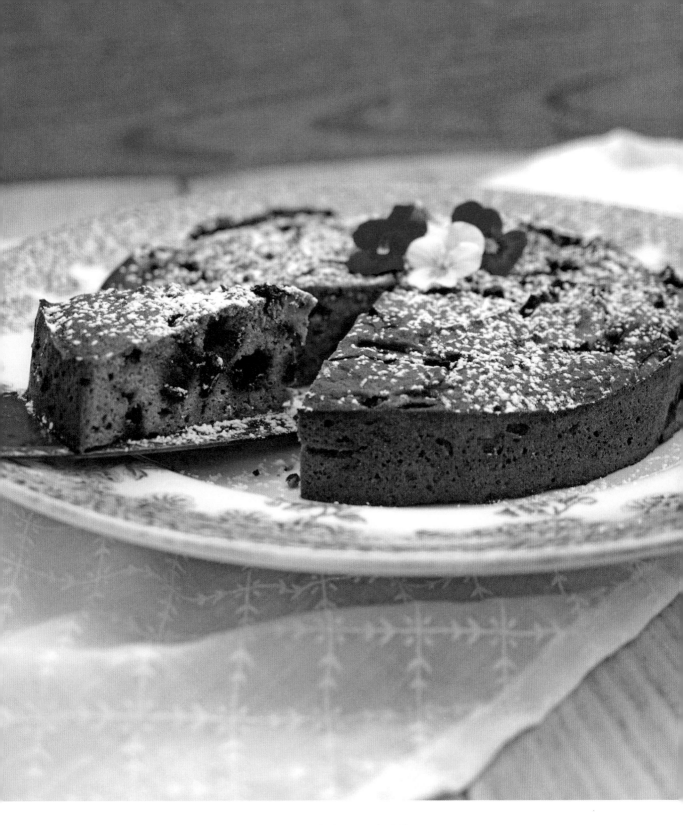

Strawberry rounds

with meringue

2 egg whites
1 scant oz (25g) low-calorie
   sweetener such as stevia
pinch of salt
1oz (30g) ground almonds
½ tsp vanilla powder
1 tsp locust bean gum
8 strawberries

Preheat the oven to 325°F (160°C). Line a baking sheet with parchment paper. Place 1 egg white in a bowl over hot water with ½oz (15g) of sweetener and the salt. Beat until stiff. Fold in the almonds, vanilla, and locust bean gum. Shape 4 balls and press flat on the baking sheet. Bake in the center of the oven for 15–20 minutes. Beat the other egg white with ¼oz (10g) sweetener over the bain-marie until stiff. Halve the strawberries and put these and the meringue on top of each cooked disc and cook for 15 minutes.

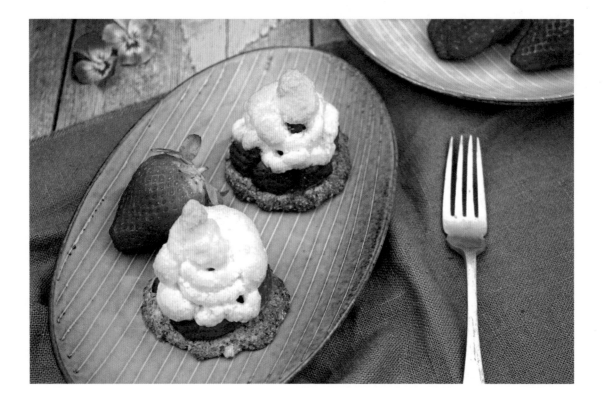

At home	At work	Serves	Kcal	Protein	Carbs	Fat
20 + 35 mins	0 min	4	80	4g	2g	4g

Low-carb cookies
with almonds

1 egg
1¾oz (50g) almond butter
1oz (30g) low-calorie
  sweetener such as stevia
2½oz (75g) ground almonds

Preheat the oven to 375°F (190°C). Line a baking sheet with parchment paper. Beat the egg in a bowl until foamy, then stir in the almond butter and sweetener. Add the ground almonds and combine everything. Use a teaspoon to make approximately 15 little blobs of mixture on the parchment paper. Bake the cookies in the center of the oven for 10—15 minutes, until they are pale gold in color. Remove from the sheet and leave to cool on a wire rack. Store in a container.

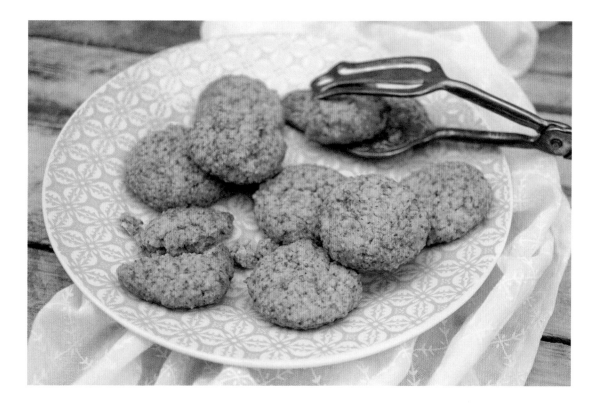

At home	At work	Serves	Kcal	Protein	Carbs	Fat
10 + 15 mins	0 min	15	65	2g	1g	4g

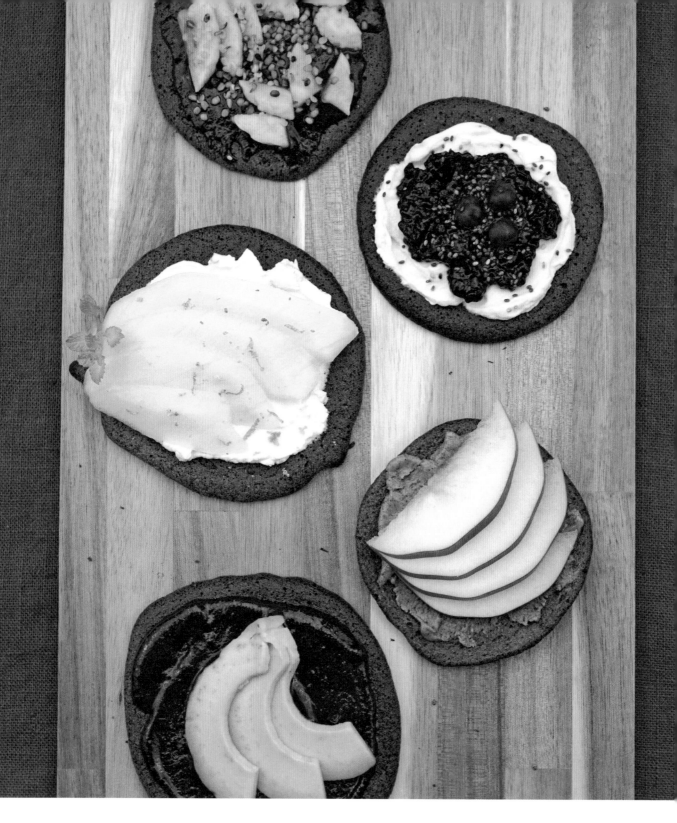

Chocolate "oopsies"
with toppings

FOR THE OOPSIES
2 eggs
salt
1¼oz (40g) full-fat cream cheese
½oz (15g) raw cocoa powder
dash of agave syrup
cream cheese, plain Greek
    yogurt, or other spread
seeds and fruits, cut into
    bite-sized pieces (optional)

Preheat the oven to 375°F (190°C). Line 2 baking sheets with parchment paper. Separate the eggs. In a bowl, beat the egg whites with a pinch of salt until stiff. Combine the egg yolks with the cream cheese, cocoa, agave syrup, and an extra pinch of salt. Fold in the beaten egg whites. From this mixture, create 10 discs on the sheets—not too close together, otherwise the oopsies will merge. Bake in the center of the oven for 10–15 minutes. Leave to cool and pack up in a container. Put the cream cheese, yogurt, or spread and seeds and fruits, if using, into containers.

At home	At work	Serves	Kcal	Protein	Carbs	Fat
15 + 5 mins	0 min	10	30	2g	1g	2g

CINNAMON SPREAD
1¾oz (50g) almond butter
½ tsp ground cinnamon
½ tsp vanilla powder
1 tsp agave syrup
grated nutmeg

Place all the ingredients in a blender beaker and use a hand-held blender to process everything to a smooth purée. Transfer the cinnamon spread to a jar and seal. Store the spread in the refrigerator, where it will keep for up to 10 days.

At home	At work	Serves	Kcal	Protein	Carbs	Fat
5 mins	0 min	5	70	2g	2g	6g

CHOCO HEMP CREAM
2oz (60g) coconut oil
¾oz (20g) cocoa powder
1oz (30g) hulled hemp seeds
agave syrup, to taste

Melt the coconut oil in a pan over low heat. Put the oil into a blender beaker with the cocoa and hemp seeds, and use a hand-held blender to process to a creamy consistency. Sweeten the cream to taste with agave syrup, transfer to a jar, and leave to cool. Close the jar and store in a cold place. The cream will keep in the refrigerator for at least 1 week.

At home	At work	Serves	Kcal	Protein	Carbs	Fat
10 mins	0 min	10	80	2g	1g	7g

Coconut waffles

with icing sugar substitute and berries

1oz (30g) butter
1 tbsp coconut oil
2 eggs
2oz (60g) plain Greek yogurt
   (thick)
3 heaped tbsp coconut
   protein powder
1 level tsp cream of tartar
some low-carb confectioner's
   sugar substitute
fruits (optional)

ALSO
waffle iron

Melt the butter and coconut oil in a pan over low heat. Whisk the eggs in a bowl. Add the yogurt, butter, and coconut oil, and stir everything well. Mix in the protein powder and cream of tartar. If the mixture is too thick, stir in an additional 1–2 tablespoons water to create a smooth, thick batter.

Preheat the waffle iron. For each waffle, put a ladle of batter onto the waffle iron and cook until golden brown. Leave the waffles to cool on a wire rack and pack into containers.

AT WORK—Dust the waffles with confectioner's sugar substitute and top with fruit, if using.

OUR TIP—If you like, you can create several portions of the batter at home, then take those to work along with your waffle iron. Freshly cooked waffles are always the best!

At home	At work	Serves	Kcal	Protein	Carbs	Fat
15 mins	1 min	2	382	35g	4g	24g

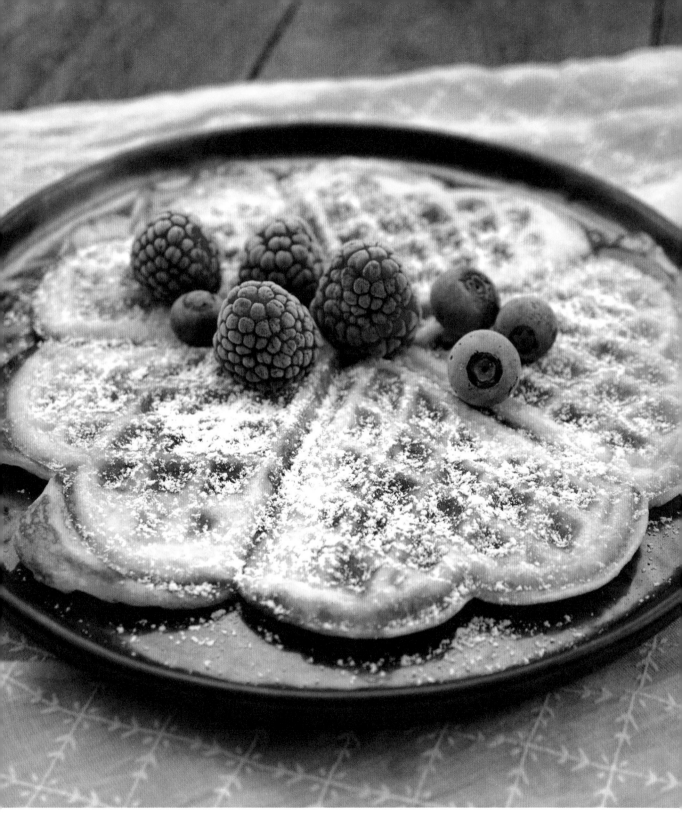

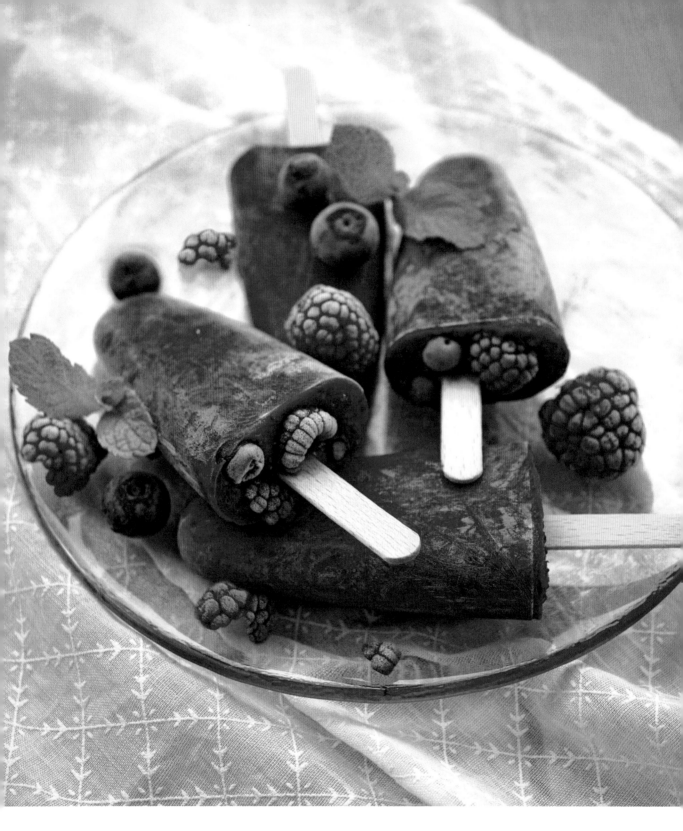

Frozen berries
ice pops

1 tbsp yogurt
5fl oz (150ml) milk
3½oz (100g) mixed berries
   (fresh or frozen)
low-calorie sweetener such
   as stevia, to taste
1 tbsp chia seeds

ALSO
6 ice pop molds
6 wooden freezer pop sticks

Put the yogurt, milk, and about 2½oz (75g) of berries (frozen berries do not have to be thawed) into a food processor and blend until smooth. Add the remaining berries to the purée and sweeten to taste with the sweetener.

Pour the purée into an airtight and leakproof container and close. Store in the refrigerator until you are ready to use.

AT WORK——Stir the chia seeds into the berry mixture. Pour the cold mix into the ice pop molds and insert 1 wooden stick into each. They will need at least 2 hours in the freezer before they are ready.

If you have a short commute you can prepare and freeze the ice pops at home. Be careful when transporting them, and be sure to put them back into the freezer as soon as you reach your destination.

At home	At work	Serves	Kcal	Protein	Carbs	Fat
5 mins	5 + 120 mins	6	30	2g	2g	1g

Pecan candies
with coconut

1½oz (45g) pecans (plus
    6 pecans to decorate)
1 tbsp coconut oil
1¼oz (40g) dates, pitted
½ tsp vanilla powder

Finely grind the pecans in a food processor. Melt the coconut oil in a small pan over low heat. Add the dates, vanilla, and melted coconut oil to the ground nuts and process everything together until you achieve a fine consistency.

Use your hands to shape the nut mixture into a ball and place this on a sheet of parchment paper. Lay a second sheet of parchment paper on top and use a rolling pin to roll the mixture out into a rectangle approximately ½in (1cm) thick. Use a knife or cookie cutter to cut or stamp out squares measuring roughly 1½ x 1½in (3 x 3cm).

Place 1 pecan nut on each square and press it in slightly. Let the candies firm up in the refrigerator. Store in a container until ready to eat. The pecan candies will keep for at least 1 week in the refrigerator.

At home	At work	Serves	Kcal	Protein	Carbs	Fat
10 mins	0 min	6	100	1g	5g	8g

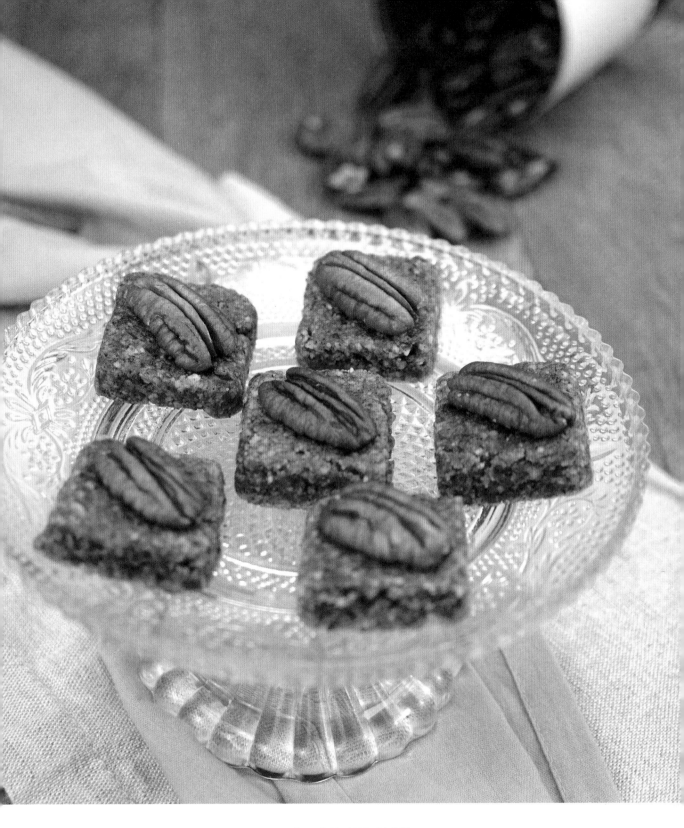

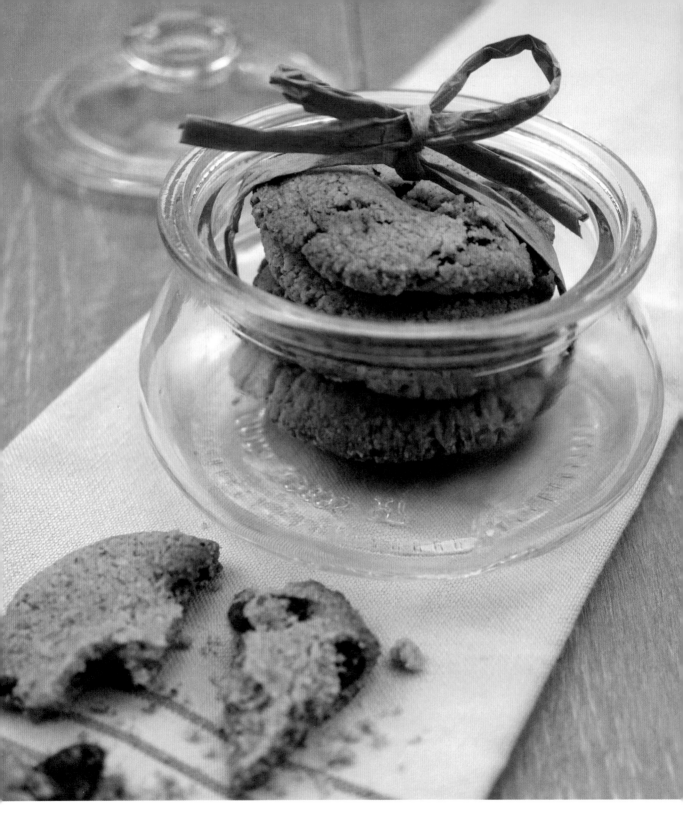

Cinnamon cookies
with raisins

4½oz (125g) ground almonds
½ tsp baking soda
½ vanilla bean
1 tsp ground cinnamon
1–2 tsp low-calorie sweetener
  such as stevia
2oz (60g) soft butter
1 tbsp raisins

Preheat the oven to 375°F (190°C). Line a baking sheet with parchment paper.

Put the almonds and baking soda in a bowl. Cut open the vanilla bean lengthwise and scrape out the seeds with a small knife.

Add the vanilla seeds, cinnamon, sweetener, and butter to the almond mixture and mix together well. Finally, mix in the raisins.

Create 12 balls from the mixture, place these on the parchment paper, and press flat. Bake the cookies in the center of the oven for 10–15 minutes, until golden. Remove from the sheet and leave to cool on a wire rack. The cinnamon cookies will keep for several days stored in an airtight container.

At home	At work	Serves	Kcal	Protein	Carbs	Fat
10 + 15 mins	0 min	12	110	3g	2g	10g

Index

A
Almond milk 22
APPLE
    Apple and carrot salad 83
    Apple and orange muffins 168
    Apple cinnamon slices 164
    Cucumber shake 26
    Yogurt muesli 44
Apricot slices 164
Asian noodle soup 139
AVOCADO
    Chicken kebabs 135
    Choco chia bowl 36
    Chocolate pudding 47
    Chocolate smoothie 24
    Cucumber power 95
    Green smoothie bowl 32
    Grilled avocado with salad 119
    Rainbow rolls 140
    Salad wraps with shrimp 151
    Strawberry bowl 48

B
BANANA
    Choco chia bowl 36
    Chocolate smoothie 24
    Green smoothie bowl 32
    Orange shake 27
BARS
    Low-carb energy bars 160
    Sesame bars 161
bean salad, Bell pepper and 91
BEEF
    Asian noodle soup 139
    Beef strips 136
    Meatballs with peas 143
Beet dip 63
Beluga lentil salad 99
BERRIES
    Berry slices 164
    Blueberry vanilla cake 172

Blueberry vanilla spread 54
Chia breakfast bowl 35
Chia pudding with berry purée 43
Choco chia bowl 36
Coconut bowl 31
Frozen berries 181
Green smoothie bowl 32
Raspberry chia spread 55
Red lentil salad 100
Blood sugar 10–11
BOK CHOY
    Beef strips 136
BOWLS
    Choco chia bowl 36
    Chia breakfast bowl 35
    Coconut bowl 31
    Green smoothie bowl 32
    Strawberry bowl 48
BREADS & BUNS
    Buttermilk rolls 76
    Cottage baguette 67
    Fitness baguette 78
    Low-carb rolls 77
    Nut bread 71
    Spelt and hemp bread 72
    Walnut bread 75
BROCCOLI
    Asian noodle soup 139
    Beluga lentil salad 99
    Life-enhancing soup 131
Buttermilk rolls 76

C
candies, Pecan 182
CAPE GOOSEBERRIES
    Kale and spinach salad 103
CARROTS
    Apple and carrot salad 83
    Asian noodle soup 139
    Beef strips 136

Bell pepper boats 104
Carrot and cucumber noodles 84
Chickpea pasta salad 107
Kimchi 96
Life-enhancing soup 131
Omelet rolls 112
Rainbow rolls 140
Cashew butter 56
Cashew citrus cream 59
CAULIFLOWER
    Cauliflower egg muffin 111
    Teriyaki chicken 144
CELERY
    Pumpkin soup 120
    Tuna and egg salad 156
Chia breakfast bowl 35
Chia pick-me-up 49
Chia pudding with berry purée 43
CHICKEN
    Chicken kebabs 135
    Chicken stock 128
    Chicory salad 132
    Life-enhancing soup 131
    Rainbow rolls 140
    Teriyaki chicken 144
Chicken stock 128
CHICKPEAS
    Chickpea pasta salad 107
    Kale and spinach salad 103
Chicory salad 132
CHINESE CABBAGE
    Kimchi 96
    Teriyaki chicken 144
CHOCOLATE
    Choco chia bowl 36
    Choco hemp cream 177
    Chocolate "oopsies" 177
    Chocolate pudding 47
    Chocolate smoothie 24
    Cream-filled sandwich cookie 167

CHUTNEY
Pan-fried shrimp 148
Cinnamon cookies 185
Cinnamon spread 177
COCONUT
Apple and orange muffins 168
Apple cinnamon slices 164
Chia breakfast bowl 35
Cottage baguette 67
Coconut bowl 31
Coconut muesli 50
Coconut waffles 178
Energy balls 163
Fitness baguette 78
Low-carb energy bars 160
Low-carb rolls 77
Mini muffins 171
Revitalizing muesli 51
COOKIES
Cinnamon cookies 185
Cream-filled sandwich cookie 167
Low-carb cookies 175
Cottage baguette 67
CUCUMBER
Beef strips 136
Carrot and cucumber noodles 84
Cucumber power 95
Cucumber radish quark 60
Cucumber shake 26
Grilled avocado with salad 119
Pan-fried shrimp 148
Rainbow rolls 140
Salad wraps with shrimp 151
Tomato and mozzarella kebabs 124

D
DATES
Apricot slices 164
Berry slices 164
Chocolate pudding 47
Low-carb energy bars 160
Pecan candies 182
Plum and cocoa slices 164
Sesame bars 161
dips, Three kinds 63
DRINKS
Almond milk 22
Chocolate smoothie 24

Cucumber shake 26
Mandarin citrus drink 29
Mango lassi 28
Orange shake 27
Strawberry chia smoothie 25

E
EGGS
Blueberry vanilla cake 172
Cauliflower egg muffin 111
Chocolate "oopsies" 177
Coconut waffles 178
Cottage baguette 67
Cream-filled sandwich cookie 167
Fitness baguette 78
Low-carb cookies 175
Mini muffins 171
Nut bread 71
Omelet rolls 112
"Oopsies" 68
Spinach wraps 147
Tuna and egg salad 156
Walnut bread 75
Zucchini lasagna 115
Energy balls 163
energy bars, Low-carb 160

F
FENNEL
Beluga lentil salad 99
Fish cakes 152
Tuna and egg salad 156
FETA
Bell pepper and bean salad 91
Beluga lentil salad 99
Fish cakes 152
Fish platter 155
Fitness baguette 78
Fruit slices 164

G
GOAT CHEESE
Fish platter 155
Goat cheese spread 64
GREEK YOGURT
Chia pick-me-up 49
Chicken kebabs 135
Coconut waffles 178
Cream-filled sandwich cookie 167

Cucumber radish quark 60
Fitness baguette 78
Lime mandarin quark 40
Nut bread 71
Papaya pear yogurt 39
Tomato and mozzarella kebabs 124
Yogurt muesli 44
Green smoothie bowl 32
Grilled avocado with salad 119

I
ICE POPS
Frozen berries 181

K
Kale and spinach salad 103
KEBABS
Chicken kebabs 135
Tomato and mozzarella kebabs 124
Kimchi 96
KIWI
Chia pick-me-up 49
Chia breakfast bowl 35
Coconut bowl 31

L
lasagna, Zucchini 115
lassi, Mango 28
LENTILS
Beluga lentil salad 99
Red lentil salad 100
Life-enhancing soup 131
Lime mandarin quark 40
Low-carb cookies 175
Low-carb energy bars 160
low carb exchange 14–15
Low-carb rolls 77

M
Mandarin citrus drink 29
MANDARIN ORANGES
Lime mandarin quark 40
Mandarin citrus drink 29
MANGO
Chia breakfast bowl 35
Coconut bowl 31
Mango lassi 28
Pan-fried shrimp 148
Strawberry bowl 48

MEATBALLS & PATTIES
    Fish cakes 152
    Meatballs with peas 143
Mini muffins 171
MOZZARELLA
    Squash salad 87
    Tomato and mozzarella kebabs 124
MUESLI
    Coconut muesli 50
    Revitalizing muesli 51
    Yogurt muesli 44
MUFFINS
    Apple and orange muffins 168
    Cauliflower egg muffin 111
Multicolored salad 88

N
NOODLES
    Asian noodle soup 139
    Beef strips 136
    Carrot and cucumber noodles 84
    Rainbow rolls 140
    Vegetable noodle soup 123
    Zucchini pasta salad 108
Nut bread 71

O
OATS
    Berry slices 164
    Revitalizing muesli 51
    Sesame bars 161
    Yogurt muesli 44
Omelet rolls 112
"Oopsies" 68
ORANGE
    Apple and carrot salad 83
    Apple and orange muffins 168
    Cashew citrus cream 59
    Chicory salad 132
    Choco chia bowl 36
    Fish cakes 152
    Kale and spinach salad 103
    Mandarin citrus drink 29
    Multicolored salad 88
    Orange shake 27
    Pumpkin soup 120
    Yogurt muesli 44

P
Pan-fried shrimp 148
Papaya pear yogurt 39
Pecan candies 182
PEAR
    Fish cakes 152
    Papaya pear yogurt 39
PEPPERS
    Bell pepper and bean salad 91
    Bell pepper boats 104
    Chickpea pasta salad 107
    Life-enhancing soup 131
    Multicolored salad 88
    Omelet rolls 112
    Rainbow rolls 140
    Red lentil salad 100
    Teriyaki chicken 144
    Tuna and egg salad 156
    Tomato and mozzarella kebabs 124
    Vegetable noodle soup 123
    Zucchini pasta salad 108
PINEAPPLE
    Coconut bowl 31
    Pan-fried shrimp 148
Plum and cocoa slices 164
PUMPKIN
    Pumpkin soup 120
    Squash salad 87
    Vegetable noodle soup 123

Q
QUINOA
    Apple and orange muffins 168
    Kale and spinach salad 103
    Multicolored salad 88

R
RADISHES
    Cucumber radish quark 60
    Meatballs with peas 143
    Salad wraps with shrimp 151
    Tomato salad with cottage cheese 92
    Tuna and egg salad 156
RED CABBAGE
    Multicolored salad 88
    Rainbow rolls 140
    Vegetable noodle soup 123
Red lentil salad 100

Revitalizing muesli 51
RICE NOODLES
    Beef strips 136
ROMAINE LETTUCE
    Apple and carrot salad 83
    Carrot and cucumber noodles 84

S
SALADS
    Bell pepper and bean salad 91
    Beluga lentil salad 99
    Chicory salad 132
    Chicken kebabs 135
    Chickpea pasta salad 107
    Grilled avocado with salad 119
    Kale and spinach salad 103
    Multicolored salad 88
    Pan-fried shrimp 148
    Red lentil salad 100
    Salad wraps with shrimp 151
    Squash salad 87
    Tomato salad with cottage cheese 92
    Tuna and egg salad 156
    Zucchini pasta salad 108
SALMON
    Fish cakes 152
    Fish platter 155
    Spinach wraps 147
Sesame bars 161
SHRIMP
    Pan-fried shrimp 148
    Salad wraps with shrimp 151
SMOOTHIES
    Chocolate smoothie 24
    Strawberry chia smoothie 25
SOUP
    Asian noodle soup 139
    Life-enhancing soup 131
    Pumpkin soup 120
    Vegetable noodle soup 123
SOY DRINK
    Chia pick-me-up 49
    Cucumber shake 26
SPELT
    Apple and orange muffins 168
    Buttermilk rolls 76
    Energy balls 163
    Papaya pear yogurt 39
    Spelt and hemp bread 72

SPINACH
Green smoothie bowl 32
Kale and spinach salad 103
Red lentil salad 100
Spinach wraps 147
Stuffed mushrooms 116
SPREADS
Beet dip 63
Blueberry vanilla spread 54
Cashew butter 56
Cashew citrus cream 59
Choco hemp cream 177
Cinnamon spread 177
Cucumber radish quark 60
Raspberry chia spread 55
Tomato dip 63
Tuna dip 63
SPROUTS & SHOOTS
Bell pepper and bean salad 91
Asian noodle soup 139
Chicory salad 132
Chicken kebabs 135
Cucumber radish quark 60
Squash salad 87
STRAWBERRIES
Strawberry bowl 48
Strawberry chia smoothie 25
Strawberry rounds 174
Stuffed mushrooms 116
SUGAR SNAP PEAS
Meatballs with peas 143
Rainbow rolls 140
SWEET POTATO
Meatballs with peas 143

T
Teriyaki chicken 144
TOMATOES
Bell pepper and bean salad 91
Bell pepper boats 104
Beluga lentil salad 99
Goat cheese spread 64
Grilled avocado with salad 119
Multicolored salad 88
Omelet rolls 112
Salad wraps with shrimp 151
Tomato and mozzarella kebabs 124
Tomato dip 63
Tomato salad with cottage cheese 92
Zucchini lasagna 115
Zucchini pasta salad 108
TUNA
Tuna and egg salad 156
Tuna dip 63

W
WAFFLES
Coconut waffles 178
Walnut bread 75
WRAPS
Salad wraps with shrimp 151
Spinach wraps 147

Y
YOGURT
Chia pudding with berry purée 43
Chicken kebabs 135

Chickpea pasta salad 107
Frozen berries 181
Grilled avocado with salad 119
Mango lassi 28
Meatballs with peas 143
Red lentil salad 100
Salad wraps with shrimp 151
Strawberry bowl 48
Strawberry chia smoothie 25
Tuna and egg salad 156
Walnut bread 75
Yogurt muesli 44

Z
ZUCCHINI
Red lentil salad 100
Stuffed mushrooms 116
Vegetable noodle soup 123
Zucchini lasagna 115
Zucchini pasta salad 108

About the authors

We love healthy eating and have run a large food website discussing low-carb nutrition for several years. At this website, lowcarbrezepte.org, you will find lots of delicious recipes, interesting contributions, and tips about the low-carb diet. We are passionate about creating new and delicious low-carb recipe ideas. And when it comes to photographing the food, we believe in taking pictures that reflect how the dishes will actually be eaten.

Our recipes contain plenty of healthy ingredients to introduce variety to the snacks and meals you eat when you are on the go. We love real food and work mainly with ingredients that are unprocessed and good for our bodies. Our low-carb dishes are easy to digest, which means that after lunch you can continue working at your very best, without any dips in concentration—the great thing about these low-carb recipes is that they don't make you sluggish and weary after eating and you won't get that craving to have a catnap under your desk.

The *Low Carb on the Go* cookbook is designed for anyone wanting to follow a low-carb diet. The consumption of healthy, complex carbohydrates is crucial for well-functioning organs and vital for our health and well-being. We also want to encourage you to incorporate your own ideas. There's more than one way to approach things. Each of us has our own ideas and preferences—and that is exactly as it should be. For that reason, a recipe should never be regarded as set in stone, and there is no need to follow everything to the letter. You can and should adapt and improve the recipes according to your own preferences.

Ideally, the low-carb approach will shape your nutritional intake in the long term and become a natural choice, rather than being a short-term diet in which you consciously avoid bad carbohydrates such as sugar, white flour, fast food, pre-prepared products, and too many pastries, baked goods, and other unhealthy foods. Look after yourself by providing your body with healthy foods.

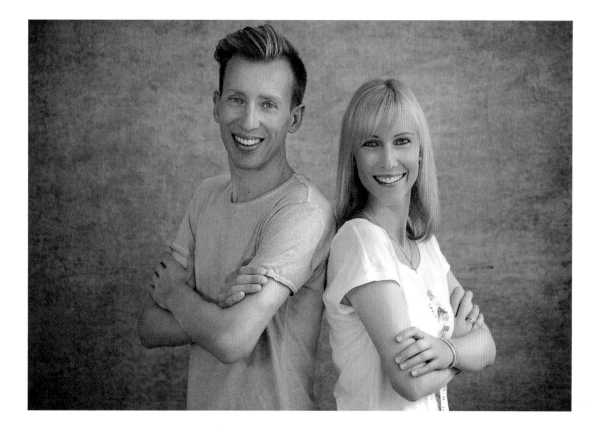

One final useful tip: treat yourself now and again to a "break" from the low-carb approach. Completely avoiding all bad ingredients rarely achieves the desired effect. Every so often, you should be able to choose a dish that doesn't entirely meet the low-carb rules. Choose your treat thoughtfully and enjoy every mouthful, then you can continue with your low-carb diet.

This way, you won't end up feeling like you have to completely miss out, or that certain foods are banned.

We hope you really enjoy our recipes.

Sandra and Mirco Stupning

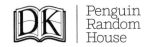

Text and photography Sandra and Mirco Stupning
Editor Karin Kerber
Designer Studio Rio, München

For DK Germany
Publisher Monika Schlitzer
Managing Editor Caren Hummel
Project Manager Melanie Haizmann
Production Manager Dorothee Whittaker
Production Coordinator Arnika Marx
Production Sabine Hüttenkofer, Verena Marquart
Author photo page 191 Julia Reinke

For DK UK
Translator Alison Tunley
Editor Claire Cross
Senior Editor Kathryn Meeker
Senior Art Editor Glenda Fisher
Producer, Pre-production Robert Dunn
Producer Igrain Roberts
Creative Technical Support Sonia Charbonnier
Managing Editor Stephanie Farrow
Managing Art Editor Christine Keilty
Americanizer Nathalie Mornu

First American Edition, 2018
Published in the United States by DK Publishing
345 Hudson Street, New York, New York 10014

A catalog record for this book
is available from the Library of Congress.
ISBN 978-1-4654-7454-4

Printed and bound in China

A WORLD OF IDEAS:
SEE ALL THERE IS TO KNOW

www.dk.com